Multiple Sclerosis

Multiple Sclerosis

A GUIDE FOR THE NEWLY DIAGNOSED

FIFTH EDITION

T. Jock Murray, OC, ONS, MD, FRCPC, FAAN, MACP, FRCP, MCFP, FCAHS
Professor Emeritus, Dalhousie University
Dalhousie Multiple Sclerosis Research Unit
Halifax, Nova Scotia

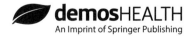

demosHEALTH
An Imprint of Springer Publishing

Visit our website at www.demoshealth.com

ISBN: 9780826165114
e-book ISBN: 9780826165121

Acquisitions Editor: Beth Barry
Compositor: diacriTech

Medical information provided by Demos Health, in the absence of a visit with a health care professional, must be considered as an educational service only. This book is not designed to replace a physician's independent judgment about the appropriateness or risks of a procedure or therapy for a given patient. Our purpose is to provide you with information that will help you make your own health care decisions.

The information and opinions provided here are believed to be accurate and sound, based on the best judgment available to the authors, editors, and publisher, but readers who fail to consult appropriate health authorities assume the risk of injuries. The publisher is not responsible for errors or omissions. The editors and publisher welcome any reader to report to the publisher any discrepancies or inaccuracies noticed.

Library of Congress Cataloging-in-Publication Data
Names: Murray, T. J., author.
Title: Multiple sclerosis : a guide for the newly diagnosed / T. Jock Murray,
    OC, ONS, MD, FRCPC, FAAN, MACP, FRCP, MCFP, FCAHS (honorary LLD, DSc,
    D.Litt, DFA, LLD) Professor Emeritus, Dalhousie University, Dalhousie
    Multiple Sclerosis Research Unit, Halifax, Nova Scotia.
Description: Fifth edition. | New York, NY : Demos Medical Publishing, [2017] |
    Includes bibliographical references and index.
Identifiers: LCCN 2017034850| ISBN 9780826165114 | ISBN 9780826165121 (e-book)
Subjects: LCSH: Multiple sclerosis—Popular works.
Classification: LCC RC377 .H65 2017 | DDC 616.8/34—dc23 LC record available at
    https://lccn.loc.gov/2017034850

Contact us to receive discount rates on bulk purchases.
We can also customize our books to meet your needs.
For more information please contact: sales@springerpub.com

Printed in the United States of America by McNaughton & Gunn.
17 18 19 20 21 / 5 4 3 2 1

To my patients ...

who taught me so many lessons. It has been a privilege to walk with you on the long road of life with MS. I continue to be inspired by your courage and strength. It was your generosity in teaching lessons to generations of physicians and to contributing to research that led to the advances that now benefit so many others.

Contents

Preface

It doesn't seem so long ago to me, but I first saw people with multiple sclerosis (MS) when I was a family doctor in a small community back in the early 1960s. I became part of their lives and struggles even though I had little to change the course of their disease. The patients taught me that what they really needed was someone who would be there when they needed help or information.

Later, as a neurologist, I was told by some patients that there was a lot of MS in their communities and I carried out studies to see if there were clusters of MS. Over those years the essential lessons I learned had nothing to do with the epidemiology of MS, but that so many MS patients in the communities felt abandoned. In the 1970s they were often told they had MS, there was no treatment, and the future would be for increasing disability and wheelchairs. In many instances, they were not given follow-up appointments because the neurologists had nothing to offer, and the family physicians said they didn't know much about MS.

It seemed to me then that what MS patients needed most was a place where they could seek help, ask questions, and relate to professionals who cared about them and were interested in them. I started an MS research center to provide care and education for MS patients and their families. It was also designed to carry out trials of new therapies and to initiate research programs that would tell us more about the patients and their ability to cope with the disease. We started with a computerized database, which recorded details about the assessment of every patient on every visit, unusual in the 1970s, but this has become a resource for research studies four decades later. It became especially useful to be able to assess the course of MS in decades before and after the new therapies for MS began to change the prognosis of MS.

Our MS Research Center offered a place of care and education provided by a multidisciplinary team, and in return the patients gave us their cooperation and support for our medical research.

It is now over a half century since I began to travel the long road of life with my MS patients. My gratitude is expressed by dedicating this volume to the patients who have taught me so much. With every new discovery, I feel a great sense of excitement about what is happening in care and research, and a tremendous sense of hope in the future for people with MS.

Dr. T. Jock Murray
Dalhousie MS Research Unit

Foreword

Receiving a diagnosis of MS does not make a glad day. There is a blank space in those words when we first hear them because we know little about MS. Immediately the void fills with the few images we have – wheelchair, drooping head, slurred words. Sadly, what we fear is all we know. Every person, newly diagnosed with MS, needs a copy of Dr. Jock Murray's book *Multiple Sclerosis: A Guide for the Newly Diagnosed*. I have been in that place and revisited an old sense of foreboding in the face of my MS diagnosis.

Finding the right sort of knowledge was a challenge for me as Jock Murray's book did not exist at that time. An armload of library books alternately depressed, unsettled, or confused me. An older book gave a very bleak outlook, and so, was depressing; a more recent book was full of undecipherable medical language, thus confusing; another had lists of so many peculiar MS symptoms for "events" which could befall one, left me completely unsettled.

Multiple Sclerosis: A Guide for the Newly Diagnosed opens the door to knowledge, a wise antidote to fear. Here, facts about MS are presented in logical sequence. We gain a basic understanding of this disease that has mystified doctors for over a hundred years. We learn a new medical language and become comfortable with a discussion of neurological disease; of current treatment and management with sophisticated disease modifying drugs; of 21st century technology; of abundant support systems; and even of positive outcomes. The old pictures are erased from memory.

It is fascinating to read about advancements made as research moves forward. Dr. Murray continues to be a key player. Promising research is presented and by nature of its vital application in the hunt for understanding of and even cure for MS, one can feel excited about the future. No longer are the newly diagnosed told there is "no treatment and no cure." However committed researchers are to find a cure, we must appreciate the importance between curing and healing.

Importantly, *Multiple Sclerosis: A Guide for the Newly Diagnosed* makes clear the distinction between these two. The book has an encouraging, optimistic outlook which reflects Jock Murray's own character. That he knows so much about MS and is still positive is a testament to hope. This has a ripple effect on patients. Hope is real.

Having this book does make a glad day, like having Dr. Murray's wise counsel nearby when healing is what one needs. Upon being given a diagnosis of MS my overwhelming feeling was, "An obstacle has been placed in my way . . . . tomorrow will never be the same." While this is true, it is not exactly true.

Perhaps one day there will be a cure for MS. Right now we stand in need of healing. Thank you, Dr. Jock Murray, for that.

Catherine Edward

Acknowledgments

I am indebted to the co-authors of previous editions of this book, Stephen Reingold, Nancy Holland, and Carol Saunders, and their wise advice from years of experience remains in this edition. I had excellent support from Beth Barry, Publisher at Demos Medical Publishing, who shepherded this project along. My friend Catherine Edward, who displayed her positive approach to living with MS in her book, *The Brow of Dawn: One Woman's Journey with MS*, kindly provided an introduction to this edition. Janet Murray, my in-house editor and supporter, assisted, as she does on all my efforts, with kind, gentle, and wise advice. She makes everything better.

CHAPTER 1

The History of Multiple Sclerosis

Before MS Had a Name

We are now aware that multiple sclerosis, or MS, occurred in young adults for centuries but it was only in 1868 that a French neurologist, Jean Martin Charcot, outlined the characteristics of the disease and gave it a name. Prior to that, most people with a progressive neurological disease were all grouped together and identified with paraplegia or paralysis. From diaries and personal papers we have information about individuals who probably suffered from the disease before it had an official name.

Early Cases of Multiple Sclerosis

The earliest case suggestive of MS was "the virgin Lidwina" (1380–1433), of Scheidam, Holland, who had a recurrent and progressive neurological condition over thirty years. She first noticed unsteadiness and falls when skating on the canals (she is the patron of the American Figure Skating Association). Her neurological symptoms increased and progressed for decades. She believed God wanted her to suffer for the sins of others, and because of her holiness and self-sacrifice she was made a saint by the Church. Her Saint Day is April 14th each year.

A young man, Augustus D'Este (1794–1848), a grandson of King George III, kept a diary for decades recording his recurrent and ultimately progressive neurological disease that we can now confidently say was MS. On the first page of his diary he wrote of an episode of blindness in one eye after attending a funeral, which he thought was due to his efforts to suppress tears, but was undoubtedly optic neuritis from MS. Over the next two decades he daily documented his progressive weakness and walking difficulty and the treatments by prominent physicians of the day, and provided insight on the treatments for neurological conditions in the early nineteenth century.

Margaret Gatty (1809–1873), a Victorian novelist and children's writer who wrote a respected guide to British seaweeds, had an episodic and progressive neurological disease that her physician thought was due to heavy gardening, using her muscles like a man. She was initially unaware that her case was published in the medical journal *The Lancet*, but pleased when she discovered this later. She wrote of her symptoms, especially in letters to her daughter.

The Description by Charcot

When Charcot wrote his definitive description of MS he was aware that a dozen other physicians had described similar cases of young adults with a progressive neurological involvement with scattered grey patches, or lesions, in the central nervous system. In the mid-nineteenth century physicians were beginning to describe many "new" diseases and classifying types of illnesses further, taking lessons from the success of botanists and biologists who had classified the plant and animal kingdoms. Some disorders were already well known, such as apoplexy (stroke), epilepsy, and syphilis. Charcot and others in the nineteenth century were able to separate amyotrophic lateral sclerosis (Lou Gehrig's disease), Huntington's disease, Friedreich's ataxia, and other neurological condition from the general group of neurological disorders. An added incentive for physicians was to have the disease named for them, so we now remember Addison, Parkinson, Hodgkin, Huntington, Tourette, Alzheimer, and many others.

Charcot and his colleague, Edme Vulpian, at the Salpêtrière, the huge Paris hospital housing over 5,000 sick and poverty-stricken persons, were particularly effective in noting groups of patients who seemed to have similar neurological characteristics. Vulpian and Charcot presented some early cases of a condition they called *la sclérose en plaque disseminée* (disseminated patchy scarring) to a local medical society, which they published in a hospital journal, with Vulpian as first author. But it was three lectures by Charcot in 1868 that clarified the disease for the medical world and forever associated him with MS. He was not the first to recognize the disease, but his great contribution was describing the disease so clearly, and naming it, so that others around the world could now make the diagnosis. As he concluded his description of the clinical features, the pathology, the course, and prognosis, he came to the discussion of treatment and sadly concluded, "After what has preceded, need I detain you long over the question of treatment? The time has not yet come when such a subject can be seriously considered."

Once Charcot framed and named the disease, more and more information accumulated about the incidence, clinical patterns, family relationships, and pathology. But as often happens, the more that was known, the more questions arose about the genetics, geographical distribution, environmental relationships, and how to measure the disease and its symptoms.

Early Therapies of Neurological Diseases

Early theories of disease centered around a belief in an imbalance in the four humors—black and yellow bile, phlegm, and blood—as the cause, so therapies attempted to effect some balance and remove harmful humors by vomiting, purging, bleeding, scarification, cupping, or other procedures.

There was a growing theory in the nineteenth century that nervous diseases could also be due to over- or understimulation of the nervous system, so complex remedies were concocted according to whether the condition was characterized as hot or cold, moist or dry, and by complex astrological measurements. Medicines administered contained such substances as musk, castor, asafoetida, valerian, garlic, oil of amber, skunk cabbage, coffee, and other "cerebral stimulants" such as henbane, deadly nightshade, and extract of hemp.

Stimulation could also be by chemicals, herbals, electricity, and various physical methods such as rough massage, horseback riding, cold water therapy, and irritating plasters. Paralysis required excitation and stimulation, so a person with a neurological disease would undergo stimulation by Galvanic or Faradic electrical charges, moxibustion, counter-irritation, wrapping in cold sheets, or hosing with torrents of icy water. Each physician might have preferred remedies, but the general list available was relatively unchanged over the century.

Advances in the Twentieth Century

In the twentieth century, research focused on efforts to understand the pathological mechanisms underlying the disease. This initially did not result in any effective therapies, but it would be an error to think that there were no attempts at treatment. Various therapies were always offered to people with MS, in the hopes that they would provide some relief, even if they could not cure. During that time, the list of therapies applied to MS patients was long, longer than today. But looking at the list today we see that few would have provided any relief, and most would have been useless or even harmful. The therapeutic imperative was strong, however, as patients wanted some kind of therapy, and physicians of course wanted to try and help their patients.

Many of the new treatments developed for various diseases were applied to MS. When the magical x-ray made its appearance at the end of the nineteenth century, it was soon being directed to the spinal cords of MS patients as a form of radiation therapy, but without benefit. Those who believed MS was due to a toxin used many methods of "detoxification," an approach, despite its risks and lack of evidence of benefit, still has some current adherents. Others felt strongly that MS was due to infection and believed there would soon be a vaccine, but in the meantime gave any new anti-infection medicine to MS patients. To remove any possible source of infection, patients were subjected to removal of their teeth and tonsils, given sinus drainage, and prescribed any medication that was thought to treat infection. The list of remedies and procedures kept growing. Finally, a young and perceptive neurologist at the London Hospital, Dr. Russell Brain, reviewed the vast array of therapies administered to hopeful MS patients in 1930 and concluded: "No mode of therapy is successful enough to achieve, at the most, a greater improvement than might have occurred spontaneously." He felt none of the treatments were useful. But such skepticism did not stop the prescribing of these many therapies and in 1936 the neurologist Dr. Richard Brickner published a 29-page list evaluating 158 different therapies applied to MS patients. Perhaps it is not surprising that he concluded that the best approach was his own treatment.

A vascular theory for the cause of MS surfaced at various times, even before Charcot, and when anticoagulants were developed in 1940, they were given to MS patients in the hopes that a drug that prevents clotting and blocking of vessels might help. Unfortunately this was before the era of randomized clinical trials, which would have shown this to be a useless therapy that caused bleeding complications.

To clarify all the confusion, the newly formed National Multiple Sclerosis Society asked Dr. George Schumacher in 1950 to prepare a report on the state of MS therapy. He thought that the prognosis in MS was not as gloomy as most believed. He suggested a means of codifying the diagnostic criteria, which became known as the Schumacher Criteria, later superseded by the Poser and more recently, the McDonald Criteria (2010). Schumacher concluded that many treatments were useless, such as arsenic, fever therapy, vaccines and sera, autohemotherapy, lecithin, x-ray therapy, sympathectomy, belladonna, endocrine therapies, and penicillin. He thought more helpful would be good nutrition, avoidance of stress and pregnancy, and moderate physical therapy. He added that no patient benefited from anticoagulants, circulatory stimulants, vitamins, and other drugs applied to people with MS. In his final remarks, he was as negative about therapy as Russell Brain 20 years earlier:

Despite a recurring "wet blanket" being thrown over MS therapies, new claims would be made and new approaches tried. In the 1940s there were anticoagulants; in the 1950s histamine desensitization; in the 1960s, ACTH and cortisone (this helped in acute attacks but not when used long term); and in the 1970s, immunosuppressants such as the growing list of anti-cancer treatments. There was excitement over the claims that the Russians had a vaccine for MS, but it turned out to be a rabies vaccine and made MS patients worse. The list of claims for new therapies grew but without good evidence of benefit, and most faded from the scene as fast as they appeared.

Fad therapies came and went regularly over the last half of the twentieth century. These included vaccines, blood transfusions, serotherapy, plasma transfusions, anticoagulant therapy, antihistamines, snake venom, colonic irrigation, hyperbaric oxygen, magnetism, bee venom, and removal of dental amalgam. We now know that these were not helpful, and sometimes were harmful. Some of these periodically come back in vogue, advanced by enthusiasts, but without scientific evidence or any accepted trials to justify their use.

The Modern Era

One of the most important steps forward occurred when Sylvia Lawry used her considerable personal energy and *chutzpah* to construct a National Multiple Sclerosis Society, which would catalyze an international movement in support of patients and research.

In the 1950s and 1960s, more scientists were exploring the immune reactions in MS. Epidemiological observations confirmed the unusual geographical distribution of the disease, with low incidence of the disease near the Equator, higher incidence in populations away from the Equator, and highest incidence in areas such as Scotland and Canada.

Efforts were being made to better classify the disease. Steroids appeared on the scene as the first convincing therapy for acute attacks of MS, supported by one of the first randomized clinical trials in MS in 1960. Early MS clinics were appearing in Montreal, Newcastle, and Atlanta. Diets became popular and the most popular was the diet developed by Dr. Roy Swank in Montreal. He was convinced lipids were responsible for MS and although the diet was complex, the essential goal was to lower fats in the diet. Many other diets followed, and although many were even more complex, they usually incorporated the lowering of animal fats. Diets such as elimination diets, low-gluten diet, MacDougall diet, Shatin diet, Evers diet, and so many others, have found little acceptance by most MS experts because of a lack of scientific evidence of benefit from randomized trials.

Although much was being learned, neurologists were generally negative about the treatments available. They also had a depressing view of the disease and its outcome and often avoided telling people they had MS, disguising the diagnosis with words that obscured the truth. Many neurologists who made the diagnosis did not continue to see the patients as they had little to offer.

The Era of Clinical Trials

The idea that therapies should be objectively assessed by rules and designs that would minimize the influences of enthusiasm, bias, exaggeration, and placebo effects is surprisingly new. Over the centuries physicians depended on observation, experience, and patient responses to indicate if a remedy was helpful. But it was evident that these observations were often unreliable and we now know that medicines and procedures that seemed to be effective for many centuries were actually ineffective. So how do we know for sure that a therapy is effective? The gold standard is to subject the therapy to a randomized clinical trial.

The first well-designed randomized clinical trial was first used in the assessment of streptomycin for tuberculosis in 1948. This trial used the concept of similar groups of patients, randomly assigning one group of patients to the treatment group and another to a similar appearing placebo or comparison therapy, with the participants unaware of who is getting which treatment.

When cortisone came into clinical practice, there were exaggerated claims that it would cure rheumatoid disease, resulting in a premature Nobel Prize, and it seemed logical to use it in MS. A prominent neurologist, Dr. Henry Miller in Newcastle, England, who had started one of the earliest medical units dedicated to MS, did the earliest randomized clinical trial in MS, studying steroids. This indicated benefit of steroids on attacks of MS over placebo and was confirmed by a larger trial in the United States. Then the American Academy of Neurology presented guidelines on how trials should be conducted in MS to arrive at convincing conclusions about how much benefit and how much risk there was in any therapy. The methodology has been continually refined since then, and is used to support any approved therapy for MS.

Beware of any therapy that does not have supporting randomized clinical trials published in recognized, peer-reviewed, medical journals, and then confirmed by independent studies by other groups.

The Modern Era of Therapy

The remarkable advances in laboratory sciences through the century and the development of magnetic resonance imaging (MRI), immunological studies, and modern genetic techniques added to our understanding of the intricacies and complexities of the disease. These advances led to the development of drugs that could be targeted toward very specific mechanisms of the disease.

In 1980 a number of meetings centered on the need for new approaches to MS therapy, better designs for trials, and collaborations that would foster clinical trials. Interferons were discovered in the 1950s, but it was decades later in the 1970s that their potential use in MS was recognized and clinical trials began. A series of trials resulted in the development of three interferon therapies (interferon beta-1b [Betaseron®], interferon beta-1a intramuscular [Avonex®], interferon beta-1a subcutaneous [Rebif®]) that reduced relapses of MS and also reduced the MRI evidence of inflammation in the brain. A different drug, copolymer-1, later called glatiramer acetate (Copaxone®), was shown to have a similar benefit. After a decade of clinical studies to demonstrate the place of these four drugs in the treatment of MS, other new agents have been approved for MS: mitoxantrone (Novantrone®) and natalizumab (Tysabri®), fingolimod (Gilenya®), interferon Ib (Extavia®), glatiramer acetate generic (Glatopa®), peginterferon (Plegridy®), daclizumab (Zinbryta®), teriflunomide (Aubagio®), dimethyl fumarate (Tecfidera), and alemtuzumab (Lemtrada®).

During the first two decades of new therapies for MS, all the new drugs with benefit targeted persons with relapsing–remitting MS, but these drugs did not have benefit in primary progressive MS. The only drug approved for the treatment of progressive MS is ocrelizumab (Ocrevus®), approved by the FDA for primary progressive MS in March 2017.

Changing Ideas

Research has clarified many puzzling aspects of the disease. For instance, MS was thought to be an intermittent disease with inactivity between attacks. We now know from MRI studies that the activity of the disease goes on even when the person has no symptoms. It was always said to be a demyelinating disease, with damage to the myelin that covers the axons in the nerves, but we now know that damage to the axon in the center of the nerve is even more important in producing progressive disability. It was thought to be a white matter disease as the inflammatory patches of damage are evident in the white matter of the brain, but with new techniques we can see there is also grey matter damage, often early, and this correlates with cognitive symptoms and disability even more than the white matter changes. The disease was thought to begin when the first symptoms appeared, but we now have a lot of evidence that the disease starts many years before and there are often signs of old changes when symptoms are first noted by the patient. A lot more has been learned about how the immunological changes produce the inflammatory damage. Many of the advances of the last few decades are discussed in the following chapters of this book.

The Future

More clinical trials for MS occur each year, and many new agents are on the horizon. As the search for therapies continues, there has also been progress in developing more therapies to treat the symptoms of MS as well. Research that shows more about the specific mechanisms in the immune system has allows researchers to develop specific therapies targeting specific steps in the immune system and even specific cells that are thought to be involved in MS.

Many alternative therapies are being studied and used by people living with MS. We hope there will be randomized clinical trials to see if any of these improve MS.

There is a long list of promising treatments under development and study so it is evident that the therapeutic era of MS is just beginning. To add to the sense of hope in MS research, we now see a great increase in the amount of research and funding dedicated to MS, and increased numbers of MS clinics, MS clinicians, researchers, and many other health professionals devoting their attention to people with MS, all striving for better outcomes and eventually a cure.

CHAPTER 2

What Is Multiple Sclerosis and How Is It Diagnosed?

The modern name *multiple sclerosis* refers to the multiple areas of "sclerosed" or hardened plaques of scar tissue throughout the central nervous system. Nerve fibers (axons) in the central nervous system are covered with a *myelin sheath*, which provides an insulating function similar to that of the insulation around electrical wires. This insulation is in segments that allow rapid conduction of electrical impulses. Plaques or patches of inflammation damage the myelin around the nerve and disrupt the transmission of messages to various parts of the body. For example, plaques that disrupt nerve fibers in the brain going to the legs could affect the ability to walk. Patients with MS often have a clinical history of episodes of neurological symptoms that are related to multiple patches of inflammation in the spinal cord, brain, and optic nerves.

Under the microscope, the lesions or plaques are seen as areas in which there is a preponderance of thickly myelinated fibers, the *white matter* of the brain, so called because it appears pale, due to the presence of myelin, compared to the *grey matter* in which there is little myelin. The area of plaque shows disruption of the myelin and some damage or loss of axons as well. There is an inflammatory reaction in these plaques, with some repair of fibers in older plaques and some scarring in very old plaques. More episodes of demyelination and more plaques may appear as years pass. Myelin can be repaired, allowing function to be restored, but conduction may be slower in these repaired fibers. Although repair can occur and may often be almost complete, the repeated myelin breakdown, incomplete repair, and accumulation of scarring lead to some progression of symptoms and signs of the disease after many years. Also when myelin repairs it is often thinner than before, and conducts more slowly.

Although a century ago MS was thought to be uncommon, we now know it is the most common serious neurological disease occurring in young adults. It occurs three times as often in women than men, and for reasons we don't understand, over the last century the disease seems to be increasing, but the increase is mostly in women.

MS follows a number of different patterns and courses, sometimes appearing more than once in the same family, more common in certain parts of the world, and more common in white people.

As the physicians and researchers seek answers and learn more about MS, they uncover more questions and more things to learn. But they are learning more, and there are more clinicians, researchers working to find the cause and cure of MS, and more research funding supporting the effort.

What Happens in Attacks of MS?

Patches of inflammation occur in the central nervous system and some of these are in areas that produce various neurological symptoms. The episodes can be brief, a few days or more likely a few weeks or longer, and in the beginning the symptoms may completely clear. We can see by MRI scans that many inflammatory plaques do not produce symptoms. When there is a symptomatic attack of MS the person might experience numbness in a limb, or on the side of the body, blurred vision in one eye, or weakness in a leg, or perhaps a combination of symptoms. More surprisingly, some plaques may develop and heal without causing any symptoms.

At first there is an inflammatory response in the plaque, with cells involved that are often seen in immunologic reactions. This has led to the understanding that the episode of demyelination, or *attack*, is an immunologic reaction of the body to some target protein in the myelin sheath, which has not yet been identified (see Chapter 3). Why this happens is not certain. There are many other immunological diseases where the body's normal defense mechanism reacts to normal tissue as if it were "foreign" material, and then reacts against it.

When the episode of demyelination settles down, other cells clean away the debris and re-myelination, or repair of the myelin, begins. As a result, the symptoms improve or completely disappear, although some subtle changes may remain. When the symptoms disappear the patient may appear to be back to normal but special tests, such as evoked potential tests, can show that the repaired nerves may conduct more slowly.

Attacks of demyelination accompanied by symptoms of MS may occur over many years. This is another hallmark of the disease— plaques that occur not only in multiple areas of the central nervous system but also in multiple events over time. Neurologists refer to this characteristic of MS as "lesions in time and space."

The Course of MS

The course of MS varies from person to person. We do not know why one person has a progressive course of symptoms and problems, while another has mild disease that produces little disability over many decades, or why different patterns can occur when MS is seen among family members.

The course of MS can be classified into four basic patterns:

Relapsing-Remitting MS (RRMS). This form of MS is characterized by acute attacks, or relapses, followed either by full or partial recovery. The periods between relapses are characterized by a lack of new symptoms, although the underlying disease process may be continuing. About 85 percent of patients present with this pattern when they begin to have symptoms.

The term *benign MS* is sometimes used to refer to a small number of people with relapsing-remitting MS who have a mild form of the disease and who remain fully functional in all neurological systems fifteen years (some use ten years as the number of years) after disease onset. This is the most difficult form of MS to "label" because it requires many years to identify this pattern. Many people with this form of the disease have mostly sensory symptoms. Because it cannot be reliably predicted early, treatment decisions are not based on the possibility that this course may occur. Because someone who appears "benign" at ten or fifteen years may not be so benign in the next ten or fifteen years, some neurologists prefer not to use the term and it is not in the accepted classification of the disease (McDonald Classification, 2010).

Secondary Progressive MS (SPMS). This pattern begins with a relapsing-remitting course, but after years may show progression over time. Prior to the recent treatments for MS, approximately 60 percent of those with a relapsing-remitting course entered a progressive phase within fifteen years. Patients may continue to have less frequent acute attacks or may stop having attacks altogether, but over the years show an increase in disability. Before deciding that a person has entered the secondary progressive phase of MS, neurologists usually wait to observe at least six months of progression, because an episode or worsening can be temporary. It is hoped and expected that the new therapies for MS will ultimately alter the long-term outcome of the disease, and delay the onset of secondary progression.

Primary Progressive MS (PPMS). In this form of MS, the disease shows slow progression from the onset, without attacks, but sometimes has occasional plateaus and temporary minor improvements. This form of MS is more commonly seen in people who develop the disease after the age of forty, and more often in men. About 15 percent of people with MS are initially diagnosed with this course.

Progressive-Relapsing MS (PRMS). This pattern of MS shows progression from onset, but later one or more attacks occur. This is an unusual pattern.

Remissions in MS

Remissions can occur at any time in the course of MS and can last for months or for many years. Why remissions occur is not known, and we are not able to tell in whom they will occur or when. Remissions are more common in the early stages of the disease and in the relapsing-remitting type. Plateaus in the course, long periods when little change is seen in the affected person's symptoms, is quite common. Remissions become less frequent as the years go on. It is important to remember that the idea of remissions refers to symptoms—it does not mean that disease activity has necessarily stopped. There is a lot of information indicating that new lesions may still be developing in the nervous system, which will lead to later progression, even though the person may feel little or nothing is changing. Being in remission is not a reason to stop therapy—the therapy may be contributing to the reason for remission.

The Diagnosis of MS

MS can be a difficult diagnosis to make. Although many patients who consult a neurologist can be diagnosed clinically on the first visit, and without any tests, other situations are more difficult, especially when a patient has recent vague complaints, shows no "findings" or abnormalities on examination, or has a symptom—such as numbness—that is common in many other conditions.

The diagnosis of MS is made by a physician, usually a neurologist, who takes a detailed history of the patient's symptoms and complaints, followed by a thorough physical and neurological examination. Although the disease is suspected and ultimately diagnosed by the clinician's diagnostic skills, two things can assist in the diagnostic process.

The first is a set of criteria for establishing the diagnosis, which were developed in 2001 by the International Panel on the Diagnosis of Multiple Sclerosis, supported by the National Multiple Sclerosis Society and the International Federation of Multiple Sclerosis Societies, and modified in 2005 and 2010 (Table 2.1). Although the terms may sound very general, the patient suspected of having MS is classified by the physician as having "possible" MS or "definite" MS. When a neurologist says that a person has MS, it means that he or she has had more than one episode or attack of symptoms occurring in multiple areas of the white matter of the central nervous system; in some instances, instead of attacks, there will have been progression over a long time, again characterized by changes typical of involvement of many areas of the white matter in the central nervous system.

When a person does not demonstrate all the criteria for MS, he or she may be classified as having possible MS after other conditions

Table 2-1   Diagnostic Criteria

Evidence of more than one area of central nervous system involvement (dissemination in "space") and central nervous system involvement at more than one time (dissemination in "time") are required for a diagnosis of MS

CLINICAL PRESENTATION	ADDITIONAL DATA NEEDED
• Two or more attacks (relapses) • Two or more objective clinical lesions	None; clinical evidence will suffice (additional evidence desirable but must be consistent with MS)
• Two or more attacks • One objective clinical lesion	Dissemination in space, demonstrated by: • MRI • or a positive cerebrospinal fluid and twoor more MRI lesions consistent with MS • or further clinical attack involving a different site
• One attack • Two or more objective clinical lesions	Dissemination in time, demonstrated by: • MRI • or second clinical attack

(*continued*)

Table 2-1 *(continued)*

CLINICAL PRESENTATION	ADDITIONAL DATA NEEDED
• One attack • One objective clinical lesion 　(monosymptomatic presentation)	Dissemination in space demonstrated by: • MRI • or positive cerebrospinal fluid and two or more MRI lesions consistent with MS **and** Dissemination in time demonstrated by: • MRI • or second clinical attack
Insidious neurological progression suggestive of MS (primary progressive MS)	One year of disease progression (retrospectively or prospectively determined) and two of the following: a. Positive brain MRI (nine T2 lesions or four or more T2 lesions with positive visual evoked potentials) b. Positive spinal cord MRI (two focal T2 lesions) c. Positive cerebrospinal fluid

Source: Adapted from McDonald, et al. 2001. "Recommended Diagnostic Criteria for MS." *Annals of Neurology* 50: 121–27 and Polman, C., et al. 2005. "Revisions to the McDonald Diagnostic Criteria." *Annals of Neurology* 58: 840–46 and Polman, C., et al. 2010. "Diagnostic Criteria for Multiple Sclerosis: 2010 Revisions to the McDonald Criteria." *Annals of Neurology* 69: 292–302.

are ruled out, and in the likelihood that additional features of the disease may become evident in time. Common examples of patients who are initially classified as having possible MS are those who present with their first symptom (since they have had only one episode, they are identified with a "clinically isolated syndrome") or those who have had repeated episodes but always in one site (thus, not multiple symptoms in the areas involved).

The second helpful aid to the neurologist is a group of tests that may confirm the suspicion of MS. Remember, though, that the diagnosis is still a clinical decision, and there is no test that says definitively that MS is present. The test can only suggest changes that are compatible with the diagnosis, and the neurologist uses this to aid the clinical decision.

Clinical Examination

The clinical examination has three major parts: history, examination, and tests.

History

The history includes not only the story of your symptoms and complaints but also your general health during your lifetime, your operations and accidents, illnesses in your family, occupational information, and other details. This often is the most important part of the examination. The neurologist often makes the diagnosis during this part of the assessment, even before the neurological examination or diagnostic tests.

Examination

To get a complete picture of your health and to better understand your symptoms, the neurologist performs a general physical examination that includes listening to your lungs and heart, taking your blood pressure, and examining your muscles and skin, as well as a neurological examination that includes examining your eyes, the cranial nerves to your head and face, your strength, sensation, and ability to detect vibration over various parts of the body, your reflexes, and your balance and walking. Sometimes a patient is surprised to have his or her feet and abdomen examined when the complaint is of numbness in a hand. However, this overall examination provides a picture of your nervous system and is able to identify other conditions that might explain the symptoms you are experiencing.

Tests

A number of tests can help to confirm that MS may be present and also can identify other problems that mimic its symptoms. Some patients so clearly have MS when they are assessed that no tests are necessary, or only one test may be used to confirm the disease and rule out other problems that might be under suspicion. The following are only the most commonly used and valuable tests.

Magnetic Resonance Imaging (MRI) Decades ago, MRI would have seemed like science fiction—a test that produces a picture of your brain as you lie inside a huge electromagnet that momentarily spins the molecules in your body. Minutes later, the computer produces a remarkable picture of your nervous system that looks much like the illustrations in an anatomy textbook. More remarkable for those who care for people with MS, the MRI is particularly good at detecting the patchy areas of change in the white matter nervous system that occur with the disease. It has become the most accurate and helpful test for MS.

The MRI examination is done while you lie on a table that moves inside a tube-like space in a large machine that holds a magnet. You will need to lie very still while the magnet sends information to a computer that receives thousands of tiny bits of information and uses them to generate pictures. These images are like slices or views at many levels throughout the brain or the spinal cord, or wherever the scanner is set. Sometimes a dye or contrast material (gadolinium) is injected into a vein to obtain more detailed pictures.

No major discomfort is associated with the procedure, no x-rays are involved, and the scanners are becoming faster, so that the length of time you are in the scanner is getting much shorter. A few people have some feeling of claustrophobia and dislike the closed-in feeling of the narrow space and the noise the machine makes. Most people can tolerate it well, especially when they know how important it is and when they have received a clear explanation of the procedure and receive support and encouragement from the staff. However, the anxiety experienced by some people can be easily reduced by mild sedation, such as lorazepam (Ativan) or diazepam (Valium) taken prior to the MRI.

MRI is an amazing technologic advance that can help in the diagnosis of many diseases and also is helpful in research. However, there are some drawbacks to its completeness as a test for MS. Because it is so complex, the machinery, support systems, and personnel needed to operate them are very expensive. The cost of the test often is in the range of $800 to $1,500—higher if more complex procedures are necessary.

Another drawback is that the MRI is inconclusive in a few patients, especially if they are at an early stage in the disease and have had only a few or very mild symptoms. Furthermore, the test does not "show MS"; it shows changes that *could be* due to MS. We must remember that other conditions occasionally cause similar changes. That is why the clinical picture is most helpful and can indicate whether other problems should be considered or whether this is a typical story of MS symptoms, with typical findings of MS on examination, and with typical changes in keeping with MS on the MRI.

Finally, although the MRI can confirm the diagnosis, it does not tell us all the things you and we want to know, such as whether the disease is mild or advanced or whether it is getting worse (those are clinical features). Also, the standard MRI does not show changes that are less inflammatory, such as those in the grey matter and in areas that appear normal. Further developments in MRI techniques undoubtedly will allow us to answer many more of these questions.

Cerebrospinal Fluid The cerebrospinal fluid surrounds the brain and spinal cord and fills some cavities within the central nervous system. A fine needle can be inserted into the lower back (below the end of the spinal cord) to remove a sample of this clear fluid for examination of cells, protein, and electrolytes; this is a lumbar puncture, which is also called an LP or a spinal tap.

A number of tests can be done on the cerebrospinal fluid, but the most useful in MS is to examine the proteins for the presence of *oligoclonal bands*; the fluid is put on a gel and an electrical current is passed through it in the laboratory to separate its protein contents into these bands. Approximately nine of ten people who have a well-established pattern of MS have bands in the cerebrospinal fluid, but unfortunately this pattern is less common in early and very mild cases. The cerebrospinal fluid is usually examined if the MRI is not conclusive but the clinical picture is still suggestive of MS. It is also an important test if the pattern of involvement is primary progressive MS, to verify that the progressive disease is really MS.

Many people have heard that having a lumbar puncture is uncomfortable, but it usually does not cause much discomfort and can be done as an outpatient. Unfortunately, about one third of people get a headache when they sit up after the test, a problem that may last for days. Lying flat on the abdomen to facilitate closure of the puncture site and taking abundant oral fluids to replace cerebrospinal fluid lost through testing should minimize this side effect.

Evoked Potential Studies The principle of evoked potential studies is simple. Nerves that have experienced demyelination conduct impulses more slowly than normally, even if they have healed and re-myelinated. Evoked potential studies measure the rate and form of the impulse as it passes through specific nerves. The only evoked potential study that can strongly support the diagnosis of MS is the visual evoked potential study.

Visual evoked potential studies assess the conduction of messages through the optic nerves behind the eyes. To stimulate the visual system, a changing pattern of a checkerboard or some other pattern causes a stimulus that passes through the visual system at the back of the brain where vision is processed. Electrodes over the scalp measure the wave form and the speed of the impulse to determine whether one eye differs from the other or if there are other changes consistent with a diagnosis of MS.

The visual evoked potential study is most useful if there is evidence of neurological involvement in an area other than the visual system, and the neurologist is seeking involvement in another area; in this case, the optic nerve. If the person has a history of a definite optic neuritis, the test is of less value, as it is already known that the optic nerve is affected.

Watchful Waiting

Uncertainty is difficult to cope with, and many people would like an answer to their problem even if it is unpleasant. Unfortunately, definitive answers are not always possible. In perhaps 10 to 15 percent of cases, the answer to the question "Is MS the cause of these symptoms?" remains uncertain even after all available examinations and tests have been done. By this time the neurologist will have eliminated other possibilities such as a tumor or a disc pressing on the spinal cord. The neurologist will know that MS could be causing the symptoms but that other conditions might also be responsible. This uncertainty can be upsetting, but the wise approach at this point is to "wait and see," with periodic examinations and visits to the physician if new problems appear or changes occur. In most instances, the diagnosis becomes clear over time. This requires patience by both the person with symptoms and the physician, but if they agree that they will wait together, the patient usually accepts the situation, having been reassured that other conditions, such as a tumor, have been ruled out. In some instances, the problem later turns out to be something other than MS, often a mild, benign, or treatable condition. It is better to wait than to be prematurely labeled as having MS on the basis of unclear evidence, especially since that may result in MS therapy being prescribed. Also receiving a label may reduce the likelihood that the diagnosis would be re-assessed.

The Outcome

When a person develops MS, she or he naturally wants to know what this will mean in the long term, relative to life, health, and family. Unfortunately, uncertainty and unpredictability are characteristics of the disease as well as of its pattern of symptoms and course. What we *can* say in general terms is that the outlook is improving year by year and will continue to improve, as the new therapies show they are better at reducing activity of the disease. Even before there was therapy to treat the underlying disease, the life expectancy of most people with MS had been extended close to the normal range as a result of the development of treatments such as antibiotics for bladder and kidney infections and better therapy for many of the complications of the disease. Newly available treatments for the underlying cause of the disease undoubtedly will change the long-term tendency for repeated attacks, progression, and disability, but we still have a long way to go. Research is proceeding rapidly and, although it will never be fast enough or great enough for those living daily with MS and its symptoms, we are heading in the right direction.

CHAPTER 3

What Is the Cause of Multiple Sclerosis?

MS has been known and studied as a distinct disease since the mid-1800s. However, the cause (etiology) of the disease remains unknown. There are many theories about the cause of MS, but the answer is still uncertain. Because the development of effective treatments depends on a better understanding of the disease, research into its cause is one of the most active areas of scientific exploration. Recent findings have brought us closer to an understanding of MS and have led to a series of new therapies and new approaches.

Theories About the Cause of MS

Multiple sclerosis presents itself as symptoms involving the central nervous system: the brain, spinal cord, or optic nerves. The peripheral nervous system, the long nerves to the body and limbs, are unaffected.

Studies of the pathology in the central nervous system show evidence of an immune reaction occurring with patches or plaques of inflammation. In these plaques there is swelling of tissue, breakdown and loss of the myelin surrounding nerve fibers, and some damage to the nerve fibers, or axons themselves. As healing occurs some scar tissue can form in the area. There may be many such scars—called lesions—widely distributed in the central nervous system, thus giving rise to the disease's English name, multiple (many) sclerosis (scars). Immune cells, such as T and B lymphocytes and macrophages— normally seen in the bloodstream—are present in the lesions and are activated against central nervous system tissue. The major questions are what initiates the immune reaction to myelin, and what is it in the myelin that the immune reaction is directed toward? The informa- tion about the immunology in MS have been extremely important because the central nervous system normally is immune "privileged" and immune cells usually remain in the bloodstream outside of the central nervous system. In MS, however, such cells become activated against myelin and are able to penetrate the barrier between the blood and the nervous system—the blood-brain barrier.

Penetration of activated immune cells across the blood-brain barrier into the central nervous system triggers a further complex process of immune-mediated damage of myelin and underlying nerve fibers. As mentioned, when the myelin is damaged there is a disruption of the electrical and chemical signals responsible for nerve conduction from the brain and spinal cord to muscles and from sensory organs back to the brain and spinal cord. When nerve signals become slowed or blocked by this immune-mediated damage, the person can experience the neurological problems in balance, gait, vision, bladder and bowel control, numbness, pain, and other symp- toms typical of MS.

Tissue Abnormalities, Infections, and the Environment: Links to an MS Cause?

Many theories have been explored as to why the myelin of the cen- tral nervous system is attacked by a person's own immune system in MS, a so-called "autoimmune" (self-immune) attack. For example, it is possible that the myelin is not normal for some reason and the immune system reacts to it as "foreign," but so far studies have not shown that there is anything distinctly different about the basic structure of myelin in a person with MS.

In recent years it has been shown that the plaques of inflammation in the white matter are not the only areas involved. Sophisticated MRI studies as well as pathological studies have shown that areas of the brain that appear normal are actually not entirely normal and show subtle inflammatory changes as well. There are also changes in the grey matter. It appears that MS is more widespread than it would seem from the patches viewed on the MRI.

The possibility that an environmental toxin or even a dietary imbalance may be the cause of MS has been considered. Although toxic substances and diet can cause other nervous system problems, there is no convincing evidence that they are the cause of MS. Occasional reports have been made of "clusters" of MS, where more cases than might be expected in a town, neighborhood, or in a school class. Such reports have triggered studies to determine if such clusters are real or simply coincidence; and if real, to evaluate any environmental factors that might be involved. None, to date, has shown a direct environmental agent to be involved in the development of MS, and most seem to be random clusters, expected in a disease that is relatively common in the population.

For decades, studies of where MS exists in the world and where it is absent (the sciences of epidemiology and demographics) have suggested that some triggering factor in the environment might be related to the risk of MS. Data from studies of people migrating from one area to another with a different incidence of the disease suggest that such a factor probably acts before the age of 15 in order for the disease process to be triggered later in life. Although somewhat controversial, this finding has stimulated the search over the last half century as to what this trigger factor could be.

Many common and uncommon viruses have been proposed as causative agents for MS over the past several decades. Many of these proposals have been based on the presence of virus in tissues from individuals with MS or, more often, the presence of immune system antibodies against viruses in the blood. Evidence was often weak as the suspect virus was often only slightly more common than in the normal population. In recent years, technology has become more sophisticated, and such searches include the use of polymerase chain reaction (PCR) analysis to detect protein "footprints" in blood, cerebrospinal fluid, and tissue even if whole virus cannot be seen. In each case in which claims for causative or triggering infectious agents have been made, further study has failed to support the claim or at least failed to provide convincing supporting evidence. Ongoing work continues to focus on a few suspicious viruses. The human herpesvirus 6 (HHV-6), a common virus that causes roseola in infants, has been linked by some scientists to MS. A common bacterium, *Chlamydia pneumoniae*, which is responsible for "walking pneumonia," also has been linked to MS by some researchers, but original claims of a causative or triggering link for this bacterium have not held up. The Epstein-Barr virus, the cause of infectious mononucleosis, continues to attract attention as a possible trigger for MS. There is increasing information about a link with Epstein-Barr virus. A study of the brains of seven people with MS showed that in plaques there are high levels of an inflammation-stimulating chemical (interferon alpha) that helps the body fight viruses, and in the surrounding tissues there are immune B cells inactively infected by Epstein-Barr virus, but no evidence of an active viral infection. This raises the question whether the virus may indirectly stimulate MS disease activity.

Rather than focusing on a single infectious agent, many scientists now believe that individuals with MS have a heightened immune antibody response against a host of common and uncommon viruses and other infectious agents, and that past claims based on antibody responses against a specific virus are likely misleading.

There is increasing evidence that low vitamin D might play a role in the susceptibility to MS. As vitamin D levels are often lower in people living in regions more distant from the Equator, it could explain the increased incidence in the same geographic regions. Some studies have shown that in large groups, those who developed MS had lower levels of vitamin D than the rest of the group. There are studies in large populations of nurses in Britain and in military recruits in the United States with information that vitamin D may play a role. Also, the lower levels of vitamin D over the winter months would explain why more individual with MS were born in the months around May than in November, possibly related to a lower level of vitamin D in the pregnant mother over the winter.

With a new understanding of the importance of immunology in the MS disease process, many scientists have shifted their view of the role of specific viruses and other infectious agents in MS away from a direct cause of the disease and toward learning how an immune system response against an infectious agent may result in a later autoimmune disease. Increased attention has been paid to the possibility that many viruses, bacteria, and perhaps other pathogens could serve as a trigger for the autoimmune process that becomes MS.

There is a lot of research into possible risk factors for MS which might influence the development of the disease or the progression. Recently it has been found that smoking can influence both. It was noted that smokers or those subjected to passive (secondary) smoke have an increased risk of developing MS, and smokers progress to the secondary progressive stage of the disease faster than nonsmokers and have a greater risk of having more disability. It also seems that smokers do not get the full effect of the drugs that benefit people with MS. It was also noted that stopping smoking did slow the progression of the disease.

In spite of years of investigation into infectious or environmental causes for MS, there is little convincing evidence for either of these factors as a potential cause of the disease. However, claims still appear from time to time in the media or scientific literature of the "latest" cause of the disease, but these have so far turned out to have little merit. However, because a possible association between MS and such potential causes could be one of the unsolved mysteries of the disease, and we know there must be some kind of a trigger that initiates the disease in a predisposed person, these areas are still being explored. Until the cause of MS is discovered, rational, careful studies in these areas are still appropriate, and we must keep our minds open to all ideas.

The Underlying Immune System Problems in MS

Research on the cause of MS since the mid-1950s has focused increasingly on the immune system function in MS and on the theory that MS is an autoimmune disease. Autoimmunity is by no means unique to MS. Diseases such as rheumatoid arthritis, systemic lupus erythematosus, juvenile-onset (type 1) diabetes (JD), scleroderma, myasthenia gravis, and others are autoimmune in nature. Many of these diseases share some important characteristics. In each, cells and/or antibodies of a person's own immune system attack and damage what appear to be normal tissues of a person's body. Most (but not all) such diseases share a tendency to be more prevalent in women than in men. (Juvenile-onset diabetes is an exception: Gender distribution is about equal between men and women and, in a few rare conditions, male predominance is seen.) All may be susceptible to treatment through a variety of routes that suppress or otherwise regulate immune function.

The evidence that the immune system is involved in MS is clear. First, people with MS seem to have clear-cut abnormalities in immune function compared with healthy individuals. These include, among other factors, evidence that specific white blood cells (T lymphocytes or T cells, and B lymphocytes or B cells) are present in the central nervous system that are primed to "recognize" and launch attacks against tissues of the nervous system, such as myelin and nerve fibers. In individuals with MS, there is clear and specific reaction of T white cells against proteins that compose central nervous system myelin. Also, B lymphocytes are involved and recent successful therapies have been directed to the B cells. Interestingly, it has been known since the mid-1990s that individuals *without* MS also have T cells that can react against myelin, but in such individuals these cells remain circulating in the bloodstream, separated from the central nervous system by the blood-brain barrier. In MS, the blood-brain barrier is broken or breached, allowing the immune cells to move into the central nervous system tissue and initiate their damaging effects. Breaks in the blood-brain barrier can actually be visualized with contrast-enhancing (gadolinium-enhanced) MRIs and other sophisticated imaging techniques.

An additional clue to the immune system's role in MS is the over-representation of cells and other immune system components that enhance immune responses in individual with the disease—so-called pro-inflammatory immune cells—and a relative underrepresentation of cells and immune mediators that suppress immune responses—anti-inflammatory cells. Most notably, in tissue from individuals with MS, immune system cells are found in active lesions of the brain and spinal cord. These immune characteristics are not normally seen in individuals who do not have MS.

Although immune system involvement in MS seems clear, evidence that the problem is *autoimmune* is difficult to obtain in humans. Actual proof of autoimmunity requires that immune system cells that cause damage in one patient be injected into a different, healthy patient and cause damage and disease there as well. Although this kind of experiment can be done in laboratory animals to prove auto-immunity, it obviously is not ethical to undertake such studies using humans, since such experiments would cause autoimmune disease in otherwise healthy people. In laboratory animals with a disease called experimental allergic (or autoimmune) encephalomyelitis (EAE), a model used to mimic the changes in MS, such experiments show that an autoimmune disorder can produce similar changes seen in MS lesions.

For this reason alone, EAE has proven to be a useful animal disease model to help understand human MS. While EAE is not MS, and laboratory animals are not humans, there are many similarities in clinical symptoms and central nervous system lesion immunological mechanisms in EAE in laboratory animals and MS in humans. EAE thus serves as a model for the study of MS, and in particular for studies on the very specific elements of immune function that might be involved in MS-like disease. EAE studies not only have contributed to our understanding of immune problems in MS but also have been used productively to demonstrate a "proof of concept" for new immune therapies that might be used for human MS; and EAE studies have led to some of the immune-modulating drugs that are used in MS today.

The Role of Genetics in MS

That there is a genetic influence in MS has been known for a long time, based primarily on the observation that MS may occur in more than one member of the same family. We know that MS is not directly inherited, but it is increasingly clear that a complex set of genetic factors helps to determine who may be susceptible to MS and who may not. Observations that suggest a genetic factor in MS come from studies of many populations around the world.

First, approximately 20 percent of all individuals with MS have at least one additional family member, either in the same generation or in a different generation, who has or had MS. While 80 percent of people with MS appear to have no family history of other cases, this 20 percent rate of *concordance* (the occurrence of disease in more than one family member) suggests a genetic link or genetic influence. However, the concordance rate among family members is in itself not high enough to support a direct disease inheritance and, in itself, does not help us understand what genetic factors might be involved. Such concordance could happen, for example, simply because of a shared environmental cause or trigger for MS. However, results from a large-scale study in Canada in the 1990s indicated that the tendency for multiple cases of MS to occur in families is truly genetic and not due to other factors such as environment or diet, and there are many other studies verifying a genetic influence.

In families with more than one case of MS the risk of disease is still quite low, and even lower as the relationship becomes more distant. In the United States, about one in 1,000 people have MS; when a family member (parent, sibling) already has the disease, the risk increases to two to five per 100, depending on the degree of relationship. If one twin has MS, the risk is 30% in the other twin if the twins are identical, but only 5% (the same risk as siblings) if the twins are fraternal. This is strong proof of a genetic factor being involved. The fact that the other identical twin has only a 30% risk rather than 100% suggests there is some other trigger involved, as they are genetically identical.

There is evidence that the genetic risk is greater through the maternal line, and the risk is highest in mother to daughter, and lowest in father to son.

Beyond the reasonably frequent occurrence of MS in more than one family member, it also has long been known that there are ethnic or religious populations in the world that are *genetically isolated*—they rarely or never marry or bear children outside their own group and thus have developed a relatively restricted and unique gene pool. MS never or rarely occurs in some of these groups. Examples include such religious sects as the Hutterites in Canada and such ethnic groups as Eastern European gypsies. While living in areas where there is a relatively high incidence of MS, these groups seem to be protected from MS. Such genetically isolated populations are of great interest in disease research—not only those that seem to be "resistant" but also those in which disease may be prevalent. Such populations most likely have a more restricted pool of genes, raising the possibility that they can be used to more easily isolate disease-relevant gene factors. Studies on genetics have been undertaken in genetically isolated populations in locations such as western Finland and Tasmania and are currently underway in Iceland where scientists hope that new clues to MS genetics may be easier to obtain.

Related to this is the fact that there are racial differences in the incidence and even in the clinical appearance of MS. In North America, the disease occurs more commonly among white people than among African Americans, even in the same community, and the clinical symptomatology and severity of the disease may be different in these two groups. And there may be differences in how individuals of different racial backgrounds respond to MS therapies as well. Pure African Bantus virtually never develop MS, although whites living in the same part of Africa are susceptible. Importantly, genetic studies of African Americans with MS may yield important clues to MS genetics. African Americans often have a mixed genetic background—a combination of original African ancestral genes and white genes that have been inherited through white ancestors since the time of slavery in North America. Through "admixture" analysis of the genetic background of African Americans with MS, Africans who do not have MS, and whites with MS, it may be possible to more closely identify MS disease-related genes, and such studies are under way. Finally, MS is seen much less often in Asians, a clinical type somewhat different from that of whites. All of these factors point to a clear genetic influence on MS even if the disease is not directly inherited.

While such information might one day provide us with the ability to predict susceptibility, it cannot yet help us. The risk rates are low even within families in which MS already exists. Inheritance patterns in MS are extremely complex and poorly understood. Large genetic studies to search for common genetic factors that might underlie MS have been undertaken in the United States, Canada, the United Kingdom, Europe, and Australia, taking advantage of the existence of families with multiple individuals who have MS. From these studies, we have learned that no single genetic factor is responsible for MS or even dominant in the MS genetic picture. Rather, there are many genetic factors that might contribute to MS susceptibility. There is no current identified single gene, and there is not likely to be one, that can be said to cause MS, as has been shown for diseases such as Huntington's chorea, Duchenne muscular dystrophy, and cystic fibrosis. However, work is underway to identify genetic patterns that might allow prediction of susceptible persons in the future.

Genetic research in MS is among the most highly technologic areas of research today. With each year, new findings from the massive genetic research efforts are being applied to the study of MS. The description of the full human genome in the late 1990s helped to identify genes that make us "human" and set the stage for discovery of genes that might underlie specific human traits and specific human diseases. The human genome map has led to efforts in the first years of the twenty-first century to describe completely the human *haplo-type* map—a description of the blocks of genes that tend to be inherited together from generation to generation. This so called "hap map" will greatly reduce the complexity of the search for disease-related genes in the human population. MS was among the first diseases to be studied by these technologies.

There is a genetic predisposition for MS but genetics cannot be the whole story. The fact that genetically identical twins are not always concordant for MS clearly indicates that some other factor, or "trigger," must be involved.

So, What Is the Cause of MS?

Multiple sclerosis is, to be sure, a complex disease that is just beginning to be unraveled. There remains no known single initiating cause of MS, and it is likely that the disease is the result of a number of related factors. While symptoms come from problems in the nervous system, MS appears to be a disease of immune system function, most likely an autoimmune disease, which attacks the central nervous system. Although the disease is not directly inherited, there is a genetic susceptibility. It appears that a genetic pattern makes one susceptible to MS but many people may have the genetic susceptibility without getting the disease. A triggering factor, or a combination of factors may be needed, but so far no definite virus, bacterium, or other infectious or environmental agent has been identified. The ultimate consequence of the immune system problems in MS is the entrance of immune cells into the central nervous system, attack of myelin around nerve fibers, and eventual myelin and nerve fiber loss and scarring. The entire process results in the failure of nerve signals to operate properly, resulting in the well-known symptoms of MS.

CHAPTER 4

What Treatment Is Available for Multiple Sclerosis?

The medical management of MS is accomplished through a partnership of health professionals, the person with MS, and the family. In this chapter, we address both the symptomatic treatment and management of the disease course.

People often say that there is no treatment for a disease when what they really mean is that there is no "magic bullet," a simple cure that makes the disease go away, as penicillin may do for pneumonia. As with most medical diseases, there is yet no "cure" for MS, but there are many beneficial treatments and approaches that will help you cope with the challenges of MS. We are in an era in which there are agents that lessen the number and severity of attacks, the progression of the disease, the development of disability, and also reduce many of the symptoms of the disease. Each year things become more positive and hopeful as we see advances in diagnosis, treatment, symptom management, rehabilitation, assessment, classification, and understanding of the disease.

Resources

One of the most important first steps in dealing with MS is to learn more about it. You need to know what you can do to stay healthy and to reduce the problems that may confront you and your family. You are in control of much that is important in managing this disease. The fact that you are reading this book shows that you are already taking charge of one of the first things over which you have control—being informed and educated about MS so that you can make better decisions and manage the challenges.

You should begin by getting in touch with groups that can provide you with information and support. The National Multiple Sclerosis Society (NMSS) in the United States and the Multiple Sclerosis Society of Canada (MSSC) are two such organizations that you can use as starting points. These organizations have up to date information sources and are there to support you. You can learn about ongoing research and important advances as they occur. These MS organizations and their local chapters have many pamphlets and educational programs on all the important aspects of the disease.

There are many books about MS. Some are excellent, and others are not. Some are by professionals who manage the disease, some are by individuals who have successfully adapted to its limitations, and some are by enthusiasts who are proposing some treatment that they are selling. Consulting one of the MS societies will help to keep a balanced view because the publications it recommends have been carefully reviewed for both accuracy and usefulness.

People with MS often hear of possible treatments from friends and the media, and it is often difficult to distinguish between those that are useful and those that are not (or those that may be harmful) and those that have scientific evidence from randomized trials to support the claims of benefit. We strongly recommend that you check any suggestions about treatments made by people other than your physician or nurse with reliable sources, including the MS societies or the books recommended in the Additional Reading section of this book.

Types of Treatment

Treatments in MS can be grouped into different categories:

- Management of the acute attack
- Treatment of the underlying disease
- Management of symptoms
- Interventions related to emotional and social issues

Management of Acute Attacks

When there is a change in symptoms over a few days or weeks, with the development of new symptoms or the worsening of old ones, the event may be a new "attack," or relapse, of the disease. It usually means that new patches of inflammation and demyelination are occurring in either new or old spots in the central nervous system—the brain, spinal cord, and optic nerves. These often are mild and cease after a few days or weeks and need no treatment. If your symptoms are severe or continue to worsen you may need to seek treatment. The swelling and inflammation in the plaques of demyelination can be reduced by high-dose intravenous steroids (methylprednisolone). Some schedules of treatment vary but a common practice is to administer 1000 mg of methylprednisolone intravenously over 30 minutes as an outpatient, and repeat this daily for three to five days. There may be variations in the total steroid dose, the number of days of treatment, and the time between doses, but all are characterized by a high dose over a short period. It is also possible to treat acute attacks with oral steroids, but it involves a very large dose of steroids, equivalent to the intravenous dose. The treatment is well tolerated by patients, although some may have trouble sleeping when they receive high doses of steroids.

Some people may begin to recover soon after steroid therapy has started, but for others, improvement may occur only slowly, even weeks after the treatment. As some spontaneous recovery is expected after most acute attacks, it sometimes is difficult to know how much was due to the treatment and how much would have occurred without it.

If there is mild numbness in a limb, dizziness, or some other symptom that is annoying but not limiting in any way, your neurologist may decide to wait and see if the problem clears spontaneously, as it often does. An attack that has stopped progressing and is improving may be allowed to clear on its own. High-dose steroids help people to recover from an attack somewhat faster, but since they might recover just as well with time, decisions about treatment must be made on an individual basis. The repetitive use of steroids can have long-term effects that include cataracts, osteoporosis, and weight gain; therefore, their use should be reserved for more serious attacks that are not clearing spontaneously. A rare but important complication is avascular necrosis of the hip that requires a hip replacement.

Although it is reasonable to rest when you have MS, especially during attacks, there is a tendency to rest too much and people who care for you will often over-encourage rest. You need some rest but there is little evidence that your MS will be worse with less rest. If you overdo rest you may actually feel weary and weak, and may stop work or neglect responsibilities when you are capable of continuing these activities. A reasonable approach is to develop a schedule that allows for a slower pace but allows you to manage despite the fatigue.

The best advice to people with MS is not "rest, with reasonable activity," but rather "stay active, with reasonable rest." The difference is in placement of the emphasis. Slow down and rest more when symptoms and fatigue are a problem or when an attack occurs, but stay as active as you can and increase your activity again when the symptoms are relieved.

Treatment of the Underlying Disease

When to Begin Therapy?

I believe there are two important concepts to keep in mind when you have been diagnosed with MS and therapy is being considered:

A. **Early is late**. This means that when you experience the first symptoms of MS, and feel it is early in the disease, there are usually indicators that the disease has been there for a long time, with evidence of changes that caused no symptoms. So it seems early, but it is really late.

B. **Treatment should start as soon as the diagnosis is confirmed**. There is a lot of evidence that the benefits of therapy are greater when started early. The object is to reduce the activity of the disease as judged by the clinical activity and the MRI activity, and preserve the brain's ability to repair itself and compensate for damage. There is a limit to the brain's healing powers and plasticity to compensate for damage, so treatment should start early to protect the brain. Another expression used by some neurologists is *"Time is brain,"* meaning the longer you wait, the more brain damage occurs.

The Objective of Therapy

The objective of the current therapies for MS is to reduce the activity of the disease. The hope is to achieve a state where there is no evidence of disease activity (NEDA). This means no relapses, no progression of disability, and no evidence of activity on the MRI. Not all patients can achieve this with therapy, so the second choice is minimal evidence of disease activity (MEDA). These concepts are relatively new, and only possible because the therapies have improved and have greater effect, especially when used early.

Disease-Modifying Therapies

We now have available therapies that offer the promise of having an impact on the ultimate course of the disease. None of the currently available therapies will cure the disease, but these medications can reduce the number and severity of attacks and result in less progression and disability over the years.

The following therapies are approved by the Food and Drug Administration in the United States and Health Canada:

Injectable medications

>   Avonex (interferon beta-1a)
>
>   Betaseron (interferon beta-1b)
>
>   Rebif (interferon beta-1a)
>
>   Copaxone (glatiramer acetate)
>
>   Extavia (interferon beta-1b)
>
>   Glatopa (glatiramer acetate)
>
>   Plegridy (peginterferon beta-1a)
>
>   Zinbryta (daclizumab)

Oral medications

>   Aubagio (teriflunomide)
>
>   Gilenya (fingolimod)
>
>   Tecfidera (dimethyl fumarate)

Infused medications

>   Tysabri (natalizumab)
>
>   Lemtrada (alemtuzumab)
>
>   Novantrone (mitoxantrone)
>
>   Ocrevus (ocrelizumab)

They have been approved in many countries, and other agents will soon appear. Each country has a system of approval, so the list of approved drugs may vary in different countries. These agents have been approved for use in MS based on extensive clinical trials and review of the evidence of benefit and risk. Most neurologists make their decision as to which drug is appropriate for a given patient based on that individual's disease characteristics as well as the patient's lifestyle and preferences. The latest approved drug has been Ocrevus (ocrelizumab), which targets B lymphocytes, and is the first drug approved for the treatment of primary progressive MS.

There is good evidence that the drugs discussed in the following sections are helpful if they are used in the early relapsing stages of the disease, but evidence for their effectiveness if the disease changes to a progressive phase or has been progressive since the start is less clear. However, some recent studies in the progressive stages of the disease are showing promise.

It is important to have a good understanding of the expected benefits of these drugs because if there are greater expectations than the treatments can deliver, it would be easy to become discouraged and stop the drugs, even though they are helping. The expectation and hope is that, over time, you will be better than if you did not have the treatment, not that you will suddenly notice yourself improving or even that relapses and symptoms will cease completely.

The MS societies have information, guidelines, and consensus statements on the use of disease-modifying agents that are very useful to the person diagnosed with MS. The National MS Society has published the Consensus Statement of the National MS Society on the disease-modifying therapies. Further information can be found on their web page (www.nationalmssociety.org).

These drugs have been shown in randomized clinical trials to reduce the frequency of relapses, reduce the development of new lesions on the MRI, and show probable reduction in progression of the disease. The experience of MS neurologists is that these drugs are important in reducing the activity of the disease and improving the quality of life of MS patients. The therapy, however, has to be continued for years, as stopping therapy causes a return of activity to the pre-treatment level.

The Society recognizes that the factors that enter into a decision to treat are complex and best analyzed by the individual patient's neurologist. Initiation of treatment with an interferon beta medication or glatiramer acetate should be considered as soon as possible following a definite diagnosis of MS with active, relapsing disease, and may also be considered for selected patients with a first attack who are at high risk of MS (classified as the Clinically Isolated Syndrome).

The first disease-modifying therapies shown to modify the outcome of the disease were interferons. Beta interferons are naturally occurring proteins that are produced when the body reacts to a foreign substance or agent such as a virus. They belong to a class of molecules called *cytokines*, the hormones of the immune system. These cytokines are important regulators of the immune response to viruses and inflammatory conditions. Interferon beta seems to "calm" and modulate the reactions of the immune system, and is referred to as an *immunomodulatory agent.*

Natalizumab is generally recommended by the Food and Drug Administration for patients who have had an inadequate response to, or are unable to tolerate, other multiple sclerosis therapies.

Treatment with mitoxantrone may be considered for selected relapsing patients with worsening disease or people living with secondary-progressive MS whose symptoms are getting worse, whether or not relapses are occurring. It requires assessment for cardiac function and has a limited total dose that can be administered because of cardiac risks. It is used less now that there are other new and powerful therapies that can be used when someone is failing on other drugs.

The whole MS community has been waiting for years for an oral drug for MS to replace the repeated injections, and the first of these is fingolimod. It is easy to take, and tolerated well, but it was noted to cause a drop in heart rate with the first dose in many patients, raising concerns about more serious complications— as this is being written a number of sudden deaths with the first dose have been reported. This will now require further assessment of the safety of the drug and monitoring of every patient for hours after the first dose.

Patients' access to medication should not be limited by the frequency of relapses, age, or level of disability. Treatment is not to be stopped while insurers evaluate for continuing coverage of treatment, as this would put patients at increased risk for recurrent disease activity.

Therapy is to be continued indefinitely, except for the following circumstances: There is good evidence of lack of benefit; there are intolerable side effects; better therapy becomes available. All of these FDA-approved agents should be included in formularies and covered by third-party payers so that physicians and patients can determine the most appropriate agent on an individual basis. Unfortunately, in the United States there are some third-party payers who limit access to some of the drugs and thus regulate which drug their members may have. Movement from one disease-modifying medication to another should occur only for medically appropriate reasons.

None of the therapies has been approved for use by women who are trying to become pregnant, are pregnant, or who are nursing mothers.

DRUGS APPROVED FOR THE TREATMENT OF MS

The following is a brief introduction to the variety of disease modifying therapies to give you a sense of the options available in the treatment of MS. The choice of the drug that best fits you, your disease course and characteristics, and your life style is a discussion between you and your neurologist.

INJECTABLE THERAPIES

Interferon beta-1a (Betaseron), a preparation of interferon beta-1b (8 million units, or 250 micrograms [mcg]), was the first medication to be approved for treatment of the MS disease process. Early studies of the drug were carried out on patients with established relapsing-remitting MS. They demonstrated a reduction in the number and severity of attacks, as well as a reduction of the number of lesions seen on the MRI brain scan. Longer term studies are showing some modification in the rate of progression of the disease as well.

The drug is self-injected under the skin every other day, using a technique similar to the way a person with diabetes uses insulin. It does cause some side effects, which usually are manageable and tolerable. These include mild flu-like symptoms after the injections, which can be relieved by simple analgesics taken before the injections. The flu-like symptoms almost always disappear with time. Local redness may occur at the injection site, which usually fades over the next week or so. Should side effects become a problem for you, your MS nurse will be able to suggest ways to help you manage them. About one in four patients will develop antibodies to the drug, and this may necessitate switching to a non-interferon drug such as glatiramer acetate (Copaxone), as the antibodies may decrease the effectiveness of the drug. There is increasing information indicating that those who started on Betaseron many years ago are showing long-term benefit from the drug, particularly those who started on the drug early in the course of the disease.

A generic form of interferon beta-1b has been recently available from Novartis as **Extavia**, which is an identical drug to Betaseron.

Interferon beta-1a (Avonex) a preparation of interferon beta-1a (6 million units, or 30 mcg), has also been shown to be safe and effective. It is administered weekly by intramuscular injection. Avonex is approved for the treatment of relapsing-remitting MS to slow the accumulation of physical disability and decrease the frequency of relapses. It has been shown to delay a second attack of MS if used soon after a first episode. This first episode is not sufficient to diagnose MS, and is called a clinically isolated syndrome (CIS). People who have had a positive MRI and one episode that looked like an MS attack (CIS) are said to be at risk for having MS. As discussed in Chapter 2, one of the criteria for labeling someone as having clinically definite MS is having had more than one attack. The MRI may sometimes show slight brain shrinkage (brain atrophy) even early in the disease, and this drug may slow or delay that process. It has the advantage of needing to be injected only once a week. It also has a low risk of antibody formation that may inactivate the effectiveness of the drug. However, some experts believe that higher dosed, more frequently administered drugs may be more effective. It is important to discuss this issue with your physician. Avonex is an intramuscular injection (similar to the flu shot) and has an injector to help give the injection.

Interferon beta-1a (Rebif) (44 mcg) is similar to natural interferon beta and is administered by the subcutaneous route three times a week, usually on Monday, Wednesday, and Friday, via a pre-filled syringe. This dose demonstrated reduced relapse frequency, slower progression in disability, and fewer lesions in the brain in patients with relapsing remitting MS. Since starting a disease-modifying therapy at a low dose and gradually increasing the dose over time tends to decrease side effects, a titration pack is available to facilitate this process. About one in four people may develop antibodies to the drug, which will require consideration of a switch to a noninterferon medication such as glatiramer acetate (Copaxone). To address this issue, a new formulation of Rebif, which has reduced development of these antibodies, may be available in the future.

Peginterferon beta-1a (Plegridy) is a pegylated form of interferon beta-1a. The process of pegylation allows for a longer half-life of the drug so it required less frequent dosing. It is injected every two weeks subcutaneously using a pre-filled autoinjector.

Glatiramer acetate (Copaxone) is not an interferon. Rather, it is a *substitute antigen* that mimics myelin basic protein, an important component of the central nervous system myelin sheath, a major immune target in MS. It is given at a dose of 20 mg subcutaneously daily by injection under the skin and is well tolerated by most people. Glatiramer acetate appears to inhibit the central nervous system immune reactions that are responsible for tissue damage and the production of MS plaques in people with MS. It has been shown to reduce both the number of attacks and the number of brain lesions seen on MRI in patients with relapsing-remitting MS, but the MRI and clinical parameters take some time to have effect. Side effects are minimal compared to the interferons because Copaxone does not cause the flu-like reactions often seen with those drugs. It can occasionally cause episodes of flushing, palpitations/tachycardia, chest pain, and dyspnea (difficulty breathing), but these are very infrequent and transient and often absent on the next injection. Injection site reactions may occur with glatiramer acetate and your MS nurse can provide you with help should they become a problem. A generic form of glatiramer acetate has been approved as **Glatopa**.

Daclizumab (**Zinbryta**) is a laboratory-produced monoclonal antibody designed to inhibit certain inflammatory functions of the T lymphocytes believed to be involved in the immune reaction in MS. It is injected subcutaneously each month (150 mg) using a prefilled autoinjector syringe. Because serious liver complications and some immune conditions can occur, liver tests are required before starting and during the course of therapy.

ORAL MEDICATIONS

Teriflunomide (Aubagio) is taken as a pill once a day, and in clinical trials has reduced the number of attacks of MS by a third, reduced new lesions on the MRI, and lessened progression in about a third of the patients. You should not take teriflunomide if pregnant or planning a pregnancy, and women of child-bearing age must use an effective means of birth control and continue it two years after stopping the drug. It lasts a long time in the body, perhaps as long as two years, so any risks may last that long. In the first months on the drug there can be nausea and hair thinning but this usually passes. Some elevation of liver enzymes may occur. Some blood tests for blood cell counts and liver function are done before beginning therapy, and then liver function tests every two weeks for the first six months and then every eight weeks on therapy. The drug seems to have an effect on MS by reducing both the T cells and the B cells.

Fingolimod (Gilenya) was the first oral immunomodulatory therapy approved for MS. Potential adverse events with this agent include novel complications such as a slowed heart rate after the first dose (patients are closely monitored for this), macular edema, and a low risk for severe infections. The slowed heart rate after the first dose can result in death so the patient has to be carefully monitored.

Results from the study of half of the patients who did the initial trial showed they had infrequent serious infections and a very low relapse rate. Patients who took fingolimod from the beginning of the study were more likely to be relapse free (61 percent) than on placebo. As experience grows, the risk—benefit ratio of this drug will become clearer. Some deaths have occurred, so at the time of this writing the safety of the drug is being reviewed.

Dimethyl fumarate (Tecfidera) is an oral medication for MS (120 mg twice a day for the first week then doubled to 240 mg twice a day as the maintenance dose). It works by reducing immune activity by decreasing the activation of T lymphocytes. Because some cases of progressive multifocal leukoencephalopathy (PML) have occurred, careful monitoring of the patients on therapy is required.

INFUSED MEDICATIONS

Natalizumab (Tysabri) is delivered by a monthly intravenous infusion. It is a monoclonal antibody against alpha4-integrin that is thought to inhibit white blood cells from getting into the central nervous system and attacking nerves. Shortly after this promising new agent was released for MS, having a striking effect on reducing attacks of MS, it was voluntarily withdrawn from the market by the manufacturer as a few patients developed a serious, and often fatal, central nervous system infection called progressive multifocal leukoencephalopathy (PML). Some but not all of the cases of PML had a history of taking another drug that would also affect the immune system so the combination was of particular concern. After a careful assessment, recognizing the risks, it was re-released, with the caution about additional drugs and for careful monitoring of patients under treatment through a restricted distribution program.

The drug has been an important addition to the options for therapy because of remarkable effectiveness in reducing attacks of MS by 70 percent and resulting in smaller, fewer, and in some cases no new MRI lesions. It is generally recommended for people who have not been helped by the other MS drugs. Of the patients who developed

PML, many were still alive but often with significant disability. The risk overall has been about one in a thousand in the first two years, but it should be noted that the risk increases the longer the person is on the drug, and in those who are positive for anti- John Cunningham virus (JCV) antibodies where the risk may be as high as eight in a thousand. The risk is also greater in those who have taken another immunosuppressant drug before going on natilizumab. If a person has all three of the risk factors (over two years on the drug, positive for JCV and prior immune suppressant drug), the risk may be as high as eleven per 1,000. In January 2012, a test for the JCVs was approved by the FDA (Stratify JCV Antibody ELISA test), which will be helpful in screening for this risk factor for the development of PML.

It has been noted that those who stop natalizumab have a return of the relapses and MRI activity within a few months.

PML is an opportunistic viral infection of the brain caused by the JCV. It usually results in death or severe disability. To avoid the risk of PML, a patient being considered for natalizumab therapy will be tested to see if the JCV is present and then, when on therapy, retested periodically to make sure the JCV has not developed.

Alemtuzumab (Lemtrada). Lemtrada is a monoclonal antibody that binds to the antigen CD52 on immune cells but we don't yet completely understand its mechanism in MS, although it is likely the drug modulates the immune system through depletion and repopulation of lymphocytes. It is given by infusion for patients with relapsing-remitting MS. There is not enough information as yet to tell if the benefits and risks justify use in those under 18 or over 65, or in pregnant or nursing mothers. The usual pattern of infusion is over four hours on five successive days, and a year later an infusion daily for three days. There are many potential side effects during the infusions and they occur in most people but only a small number are serious. It is important for patients to be aware of the symptoms they might experience. The neurologist will monitor the patient for any evidence of autoimmune thyroid disorders, which can occur in one out of three people who receive the infusions. Also, patients will be assessed for immune thrombocytopenia (about two in a hundred risk for this), a drop in platelets in the blood, which can cause bleeding. About three in a thousand patients might get a glomerular nephropathy, a kidney disorder. A number of different infections may also occur as the immune reactions are altered, so these must be identified and treated.

Novantrone (mitoxantrone). Novantrone is an antineoplastic drug that is used in some forms of cancer, but has been found in trials to reduce progression in relapsing-remitting MS patients who have entered a secondary-progressive stage of the disease. It targets T and B cells and macrophages that are involved in the immune reaction in MS. It is administered by a intravenous infusion, and this has to be done with supervision as the drug can cause damage if it gets into other tissues. Because the drug can cause damage to the heart, assessment of the cardiogram and left ventricular ejection fraction is done before therapy and before each infusion. An infusion is given every three months. Because the risk of heart effects increases as the amount of drug increases, it is usually limited to a total dose (140 mg/m^2), which is usually the amount given over about two to three years. Cardiac assessments will continue after therapy to look for any late cardiac effects. Another risk is the development of leukemia, which might occur in one patient out of four hundred treated.

Ocrelizumab (Ocrevus). An important addition to the therapies for MS was the approval by the FDA in late March 2017 of Ocrevus. All the other approved therapies are for relapsing-remitting MS; this is the first drug for patients with primary-progressive MS (PPMS). The patients with PPMS have been waiting a long time for a drug that would help them. The drug is a humanized monoclonal antibody that binds to CD20 on the surface of B cells and causes a depletion in the population of B cells. It is given by an intravenous infusion, 300 mg initially, repeated in two weeks and the 600 mg every six months.

Experimental Drugs

At present, several medications are under study and if the trials show acceptable benefit and safety, applications will be made to the FDA for approval for treatment of people with MS. This is a very detailed and rigorous process, aimed at both bringing new and better therapies and also ensuring protection for patients. In the next few years we shall see a number of new effective therapies for MS.

Sequencing of Drug Therapy

MS drugs have different ways to interfere with the immune response that is producing the disease activity. Some reduce the activity of immune cells by altering their release of cytokines, and others may prevent the immune cells from getting into the nervous system. Others act by reducing the population of cells that are involved in the immune reaction. It might then seem logical to combine drugs to get combined effects. The problems are twofold: There are safety reasons as the risk of serious side effects is increased by combining drugs, and the costs would be prohibitive. The approach instead is one of sequencing. Your physician will help you select the initial therapy that seems appropriate for you, your lifestyle, and the activity of your disease. If there is a reason to move to another drug, the selection could be based on increasing the impact of the drug, which might bring increased risk.

Vitamin D

There is increasing evidence that vitamin D plays a role in the risk of developing MS and in the disease activity. There is some evidence that deficiency of vitamin D in the mother during pregnancy might increase the risk of MS in the child later in life. Vitamin D has a known effect on the immune system and that might explain the relationship to MS activity. It has immunomodulatory function, modifying cytokines to a more anti-inflammatory profile. As a result of a number of studies linking low vitamin D to the risk of developing MS and to relapses of the disease, many have started taking vitamin D as a treatment before there is a definitive clinical trial to demonstrate a therapeutic benefit. However, it may be difficult to carry out such a large trial, and since taking vitamin D is safe and cheap, and does not require a prescription, it is often recommended for patients. There is early evidence that the MRI activity may be reduced by vitamin D therapy. The effect of vitamin D in studies seems to be greater in the white population and in women. The most effective dose is not known but many are recommending doses in the 1,000 to 5,000 IU range. The type of vitamin D may make a difference. A recent study indicated that it was difficult to increase vitamin D blood levels in MS patients using over-the-counter low dose cholecalciferol (LDC, unhydroxylated vitamin D_3) but high dose ergocalciferol (HDE, fungal-derived vitamin D_2) had a greater ability to raise vitamin D levels. Despite the safety of high doses of vitamin D (up to 10,000 IU have been taken by some patients without problems), it is reasonable to have serum levels of calcium and phosphorus periodically tested to make sure there are no serious metabolic disturbances.

Stem Cell Transplantation

There are a number of studies underway to assess the results of autologous stem cell transplantation following bone marrow suppression in MS. The method involves taking stem cells from the person, then by immunosuppressant therapy the bone marrow is suppressed. Bone marrow function in making new blood components is re-established by giving the person back their own stem cells (autologous hematopoietic cell transplant [HCT]). In the many trials underway there has been remarkable reduction in the activity of MS. They had no further activity on the MRI, no relapses, and some patients show surprising improvement. This is important, as this is a very risky and expensive procedure with a 5 percent mortality. Initially only very advanced and rapidly progressive patients were studied, so the good results are impressive as this is a group of patients who have failed on other therapies. More recent studies, following the patients for 5 to 10 years after bone marrow suppression and stem cell transplantation, have shown impressive results. After five years, almost 70 percent of the patients had no evidence of disease activity—no relapses, no progression, and no new lesions on the MRI, fulfilling the criteria of NEDA (i.e., no evidence of disease activity). This procedure would never be a practical procedure for the many hundreds of thousands of MS patients, but we will likely learn very important information that will be used to develop other approaches that are more practical, safe, and effective. It already tells us it is possible to stop the disease at least for many years, and we will see if that is permanent as time goes on. The results after five and ten years in some patients are very promising.

This is not to be confused with "stem cell injections," which have been advertised on the Internet, offered by over 350 private clinics in the United States and many in other countries, but without the necessary randomized clinical trials to show if there is any benefit.

Biomarkers

In the future, we hope to have ways to determine the risk of developing MS, the activity of the disease, and the response to therapy by tests that can be used to monitor patients. There is a lot of research seeking *biomarkers*, which are measures of biological activity, that assess biological indicators, so we can identify and monitor MS and the response to therapy. Currently we use clinical assessment and increasingly the MRI to define the level of disease activity, but in the future we hope to have blood tests that could be used to measure different aspects, and results assessed and therapy adjusted. It would be helpful to be able to have biomarkers that identify the risk of developing MS, of monitoring the progression and changes in the disease and what therapeutic approach would work best in each patient at different stages, and how well a medical therapy is working. Recently, Australian researchers are exploring changes in a pathway in the central nervous system activated by chronic inflammation called the kynurenine pathway, which may be a biomarker for the switch in patients from the milder pattern of MS to the more progressive form. Recently a biomarker, micro-RNA, has been found to be a way to assess the amount of inflammation and tissue destruction during the course of MS, so this may be an indicator of when and how to change therapy. This is a very promising area of research that could lead to more effective ways to classify patients, design specific treatment programs, and assess their status.

Management of Symptoms

The most common symptoms of MS include numbness, fatigue, weakness, blurred vision, poor balance, bladder frequency and urgency, and difficulty walking. It is important to recognize that although a wide range of symptoms may occur with MS, a given individual may experience only some of them and never have others. Some symptoms may occur once, resolve, and never return. Because it is such an individual disease, it is not helpful—and may be misleading and frightening—to compare yourself with someone else, who often will have different symptoms, a different pattern of disease, and a different course.

WEAKNESS

It is common for a person with MS to have symptoms of weakness in one or both legs. Initially this may be transient, lasting days or weeks during an attack, but in some people, weakness progresses over many years as a major symptom. Because the nerves in the central nervous system have important function in the motor control over muscles, patches of demyelination may affect these fibers and cause weakness in different muscle groups, most commonly in the legs. In some people, especially those who develop the disease after the age of forty, leg weakness and spasticity may be the only symptoms of MS, progressing slowly without any acute attacks.

It is common to develop weakness during an attack of MS, but sometimes weakness may be present all the time. The pattern of weakness can be asymmetrical, involving one limb or one side more than the other, or it can seem to be only in the legs. If it comes on in an acute attack, it is treated with intravenous steroids. If it is persistent, it is important for the neurologist to decide how much is related to weakness in the muscles, how much is due to spasticity or increased tone in the muscles, and how much is contributed by a change in sensation that makes the limbs seem more clumsy. If weakness is present, it is important to increase your level of exercise to strengthen the muscles. A physical therapist can help if you experience a lot of weakness, but if the weakness is mild, you can do an exercise program on your own. It is important to remember that any muscle can be strengthened. Just as "normal" muscles can be made stronger by exercise, weak ones also can be trained and strengthened by exercise. The muscles may not return to normal, but they will be stronger than they otherwise would have been, and that is always worthwhile.

If there is a lot of weakness in a limb, various aids, such as an ankle brace for foot drop or a cane, may be necessary to help with walking until improvement is seen. Foot drop usually is first noticed when "tripping" over your foot occurs, causing the tips of shoes on the affected side to become scraped or scuffed. If weakness persists after treatment with steroids, a referral for physical therapy may be arranged so that the problems can be assessed, an exercise program developed, and any immediate problems treated. You should continue a regular exercise program even after weakness has improved (see the section "A Note About Exercise" later in this chapter).

SPASTICITY

A complex control of muscle movements normally allows some muscles to contract and others to relax when a movement is carried out. This normal pattern can be disrupted when nerves in the central nervous system are damaged by MS, resulting in the simultaneous contraction of many muscles, both the ones that help (agonists) and those that oppose the movement (antagonists). This causes the "tone" to increase in all the muscles, the limb to feel tight, and the limb movements to be slower and less smooth. It is more difficult and more tiring to walk with legs that have spasticity.

Spasticity can be reduced by exercise and by normal use of the muscles. It is important to perform stretching exercises of the spastic, tight muscles to prevent *contractures,* a state in which the tight muscle shortens. Each muscle should be stretched fully and held for a minute (see the section "A Note About Exercise" later in this chapter).

A number of over–the–counter muscle relaxants do not work well in MS and can have side effects. An effective medication for spasticity and the symptoms that it produces (spasms, cramps, pain, aching) is baclofen (Liorisol), which can be taken in different ways depending on the symptoms, their severity, and the person's tolerance to the medication. Because some people have painful spasms only at night and minor spasticity in the daytime, a nightly dose may be all that is needed. Others need relief from spasticity all the time, and a schedule of multiple doses a day is developed. Because all patients can reach a dosage level that seems too high, causing a general feeling of weakness and drowsiness, your doctor may start you with a very low dose, perhaps half a tablet (5 mg) twice a day, and slowly increase by adding a further half tablet every 3 or 4 days until symptoms are reasonably controlled. If symptoms are helped at a low dose, the dose will be held there. If you develop side effects when the dose is increased, the effects may be eliminated by skipping a dose and going back to the previous level. Baclofen is very helpful in reducing the spasms and pain sometimes associated with spasticity, but it is only somewhat helpful in improving function that has been limited by spasticity. The level that patients can tolerate is varied and some cannot tolerate even the lowest dose. This is unfortunate as the benefits are greater with higher doses. One way to get higher doses into the nervous system has been with the baclofen pump, which requires surgical insertion of an apparatus that injects baclofen into the cerebrospinal space. It can be effective in keeping the person mobile who is requiring aids to get around, but is complex, expensive, and only available where there is a system organized to provide the service.

Tizanidine (Zanaflex) is also an effective antispasticity agent that has effects similar to those of baclofen. It is especially effective for night spasms and sometimes is effective in reducing spasticity in patients who do not respond to other agents. Its use in combination with low doses of baclofen may produce an optimal antispasticity effect with fewer side effects. It has the benefit of not having the dose-dependent weakness seen with baclofen but has the disadvantage of causing fatigue in many patients. Since people with MS already have a lot of fatigue, adding a drug that might cause more fatigue is a problem. It can be minimized by slowly increasing the dose as this therapy begins.

Dalfampridine (Ampyra) was approved by the FDA in 2010 to improve walking speed in patients with MS, the first symptomatic drug approved specifically for MS. It is a potassium channel blocker and increases the conduction in demyelinated nerves. The usual dose is 10 mg twice a day twelve hours apart. In clinical trials, about one third of patients had a 25 percent improvement in their walking speed. The improvement is lost if the drug is stopped. It is interesting to note that the improvement was seen in all groups of MS patients including those with primary progressive MS.

DISTURBANCES OF BALANCE AND GAIT

Disturbances of balance and gait are common in MS because they can be caused by changes in different parts of the nervous system. A person may notice that he or she does not walk or stand as steadily if experiencing incoordination, weakness in one or more limbs, numbness, dizziness, vertigo, or even visual problems. One of the most troublesome causes of gait disturbance is spasticity in the muscles of the legs. For some people, this is the most limiting problem of MS. Because so much of what we do involves being mobile, this problem causes the most disability and handicap in the disease over the lifetime of many (but not all) people with MS.

In many instances, difficulty in walking comes with the various symptoms of an attack of MS, improving or clearing as the attack settles down. In other instances, it is an ongoing problem. A person with MS may have few other problems except a gait difficulty that slowly increases over a period of years. This pattern is more common in those who develop the disease later in life.

Physical therapy can be helpful for gait difficulty, and a physical therapist can show you techniques of gait training, muscle strengthening, exercises, safety hints, and the use of mobility aids.

A Note About Exercise: Exercise is important for everyone, especially a person with MS. A program of range-of-motion exercises is one exercise program that you should do daily, or even more than once a day if your muscles are very stiff. Each joint is put through its full range of motion to keep it healthy and lubricated and to stretch and loosen the muscles that move the joints.

A simple exercise program that anyone can manage is the 10-10-20 exercise program, in which ten general exercises are performed, each for ten repetitions, for a duration of a twenty-minute exercise period. The ten exercises are general ones that improve overall fitness. They can be altered according to individual capacity and the need to overcome specific problems or weak areas. They can be individually designed by a physical therapist and modified as needed.

Swimming has a number of advantages, although it often is more difficult to arrange on a regular basis. Swimming exercises most muscles, and some movements and exercises can be done more easily in water because the water supports the body during movement. The water should be cool because most people with MS are sensitive to heat and may be bothered by exercises that increase body heat or by warm exercise rooms. Function may be improved just by cooling in a swimming pool. Although swimming in the ocean can have the same effect, waves can easily put you off balance.

Relaxation techniques are useful and improve the enjoyment and rewards of a regular exercise program. They involve methods of learning positive relaxation of the mind and body, deep breathing, and mental imagery, combined with alternating contraction and relaxation of various muscles.

An exercise program should be regular and enjoyable. Anyone can carry out a boring exercise program for a few weeks, but not for a lifetime—which is what we all need to do. That is why many basements have a corner with almost new exercise equipment gathering dust. Some machines look terrific, but they are not very enjoyable to use, and sometimes we think that it is the machines (or physiotherapists) that are going to make us strong. YOU do the exercises, not the machine.

Exercise programs that many people enjoy include swimming, mat exercises, walking, yoga, and tai chi, but you must think about the exercises that you would find most enjoyable and can imagine still doing regularly years from now.

SENSORY SYMPTOMS

Numbness: The term *numbness* covers many alterations to the sensory system that affect sensation, particularly in the skin. People may experience numbness, but more often they feel tingling, pins and needles, burning, coldness, or other sensations that are difficult to describe. The disruption to the sensory nerves can be caused by damage to the spinal cord, the brainstem, or the brain itself.

Tingling and numbness are "normal" symptoms that virtually everyone has experienced (a leg falling "asleep," dental anesthesia, cold feet in the winter), but these common occurrences are due to pressure, anesthetics, or cold to a peripheral nerve in an arm or leg, whereas MS affects the myelin of the nerves (and sometimes the underlying nerves) in the central nervous system. It may seem as if the nerve in the leg (the peripheral nervous system) is affected in MS, but in fact the demyelination is in the central nervous system. Numbness most often is felt in the ends of the limbs, the feet and lower legs, or the hands, but it can seem to rise from the legs up to the upper abdomen. Sometimes the numbness seems to have a level, as if a belt of numbness were wrapped around the abdomen; it also may be painful, with decreased sensation below the level.

Although numbness often is only a brief annoyance, it can cause other problems if it persists or only partially clears. You may drop things when your hands and fingertips are numb, even light objects such as paper, because you do not know how tightly you are gripping them. Because feeling in your fingers is decreased, you may need to use your vision to help recognize things that you could identify previously with your fingertips. You may have trouble identifying objects in your purse or pocket because numbness can decrease your ability to recognize a comb or a coin by its characteristic feel.

You may not realize that good balance involves sensing information about the muscles and tendons in the limbs, which is carried to the nervous system by sensory nerves. If numbness is present in the legs, people use their eyes to maintain good balance, and tend to look down as they walk. On the other hand, they will have more difficulty if they look up or around, and if they walk on uneven ground or in the dark.

Numbness occasionally is accompanied by disagreeable sensations called *dysesthesias*, such as burning, "creepy-crawly" feelings, or sensitive skin (sensations similar to those felt when dental anesthesia is wearing off). These disagreeable feelings usually improve as sensation improves, but they sometimes require treatment. When numbness or dysesthesias occur as part of an acute attack, it usually improves with intravenous steroids. More persistent disagreeable sensations may be reduced by a tricyclic antidepressant such as amitriptyline (Elavil). This medication, although an antidepressant, has other beneficial effects and is useful in many pain syndromes as well as disturbing sensory problems.

Some changes in sensation are described as pain, which is discussed later in this chapter. One of these is the symptom of an electric shock–like feeling in the back or limbs on flexing the neck. This occurs when there is some inflammation in the posterior columns of the cervical spinal cord, and the bending of the neck stretches these inflamed fibers, causing them to fire. The symptom is called *Lhermitte's phenomenon*, after the French neurologist who described it. It often is transient, clearing when the inflammation abates, and can be made to clear faster with intravenous steroids.

Facial Numbness: A common and upsetting symptom in MS is numbness on one side of the face. However, this is a minor symptom that usually clears without treatment. You might have a tingling feeling or a numbness, often described as similar to dental anesthesia, that at times can involve the gums and tongue. Symptoms around the face are perceived as more disturbing to people than the same degree of numbness elsewhere, such as the foot or hand, but facial numbness often goes away in days or a few weeks. The neurologist may also find subtle differences to various sensations in the face on examination, of which the person is unaware.

Vision Loss: Several types of vision problems may occur in MS. *Optic neuritis* (sometimes called retrobulbar neuritis) is an episode of demyelination in the optic nerve behind the eyeball. Because it occurs in the nerve, a physician looking in the eye during the first episode may not see anything wrong. Later, some scarring may occur in the optic nerve, and it will look pale in the back of the eye, when seen by the doctor through a hand-held instrument called an ophthalmoscope. High-dose intravenous steroids is the standard treatment when one eye or occasionally both eyes are affected. Symptoms include blurred vision, loss of peripheral or "side" vision, and one or more black or "blind" spots. Total loss of vision in one eye may occur in some instances, but this will usually improve with time. Optic neuritis sometimes also causes pain in the eye, which clears quickly when steroid treatment is begun. Vision returns more slowly. It is common for individuals with relapsing-remitting MS to have one or more episodes of optic neuritis, although many people never experience this problem.

Another visual complaint people with MS may experience is a vague feeling that their vision is not as clear as it should be, even if a recent eye examination indicates vision to be normal. The problem may be with certain contrasts in the visual fields, or with color, which causes a mild change that usually is not detected on standard eye tests. When this occurs, text with sharp contrast is easiest to read. A related symptom is a decrease in vision associated with exercise (Uhthoff's phenomenon), which is probably related to an increase in body heat that affects nerve conduction. Vision returns when the person stops exercising and cools down.

Some people with MS experience double vision and complain that they cannot see well. Actually, the vision in each eye separately may be normal, but the eyes do not focus together. Although it is annoying, double vision usually clears on its own or responds to intravenous steroids. It is rarely a persistent problem and can be temporarily relieved by patching one eye.

Another problem with eye control that may be experienced as a visual problem is *nystagmus*. When your physician asks you to move your eyes in different directions, he or she is testing eye movements and control. Nystagmus is a regular fine jerkiness of the eyes that may occur when looking to the sides, which usually is not noticed by the patient. Sometimes the eyes operate differently in that situation, with one having more jerkiness than the other. This causes a sensation that the environment is moving (oscillopsia) or looks double when looking to the sides. In some people, the pupillary response to light is slowed, experienced as difficulty with bright lights, especially while driving at night. Glasses with photosensitive lenses usually compensate for this problem.

All that affects vision is not MS, and you should have regular eye examinations to see if you need glasses to correct the vision changes and eye problems that occur in all of us with age.

Pain: At one time, it was believed that pain was unusual in MS. We now know that pain, in one form or another, occurs in more than half of all people who have the disease. It may take the form of an aching in muscles, shooting pains, jabbing facial pain, or discomfort from burning, tingling, or other sensory changes. The first step is to determine the specific cause of the pain. Not all pain is the result of MS, so other problems must be considered. Since pain problems in MS have specific treatments, as does pain from other causes, it is important to identify the underlying cause.

The pain of spasms and cramps in the large muscles of the legs that occur when tone is increased by spasticity can be reduced by

Remember that not all symptoms in people with MS are due to the MS, as all the problems that occur in anyone else can also occur in the person with MS.

Joint pain, back pain, abdominal pain, headaches, and other problems may be due to conditions that have nothing to do with MS and should be investigated and treated just as they would if MS were not present.

physical therapy, exercise, relaxation techniques, passive stretching, massage, and local cold. The pain associated with spasticity can often be effectively reduced with baclofen or tizanidine (Zanaflex).

Facial Pain: A type of nerve pain that can occur in the face, called *trigeminal neuralgia*, is characterized by a sharp, jabbing, knife-like pain, usually over the cheek and sometimes over the eye on one side. Although it can occur as an isolated syndrome in the elderly, it often indicates the underlying demyelinating process of MS in a younger person. Several types of pain occur in the face, including temporo-mandibular joint (TMJ) pain, tension headache, and migraine. If trigeminal neuralgia is the cause, it is treated with a group of medi-cations that decrease the nerve firing. The initial treatment usually is carbamazepine (Tegretol), to which most people quickly respond well. In those few people who have unacceptable side effects, baclofen, diphenylhydantoin (Dilantin), gabapentin (Neurontin), or duloxetine hydrochloride (Cymbalta) is substituted.

A small number of people do not tolerate these medications, lose the beneficial drug effect over time, or do not respond to them. In such cases, a surgical procedure may be considered. It usually is done on an outpatient basis by a needle procedure through the face into the trigeminal (fifth cranial) nerve. This is usually successful. Trigeminal neuralgia associated with MS is due to the presence of a plaque in the connections of the fifth cranial nerve in the brainstem. Although it can cause severe facial pain, trigeminal neuralgia usu-ally is successfully managed. It is not uncommon for the problem to return months or years after it has been controlled, but treatment can be restarted if it does.

Hearing Changes: It is unusual for people with MS to notice any change in hearing other than that seen in the normal population, but MS can on occasion cause a decrease in hearing. More commonly, a subtle change can be noted on specific testing of the hearing sys-tem, but without producing noticeable symptoms. Significant hear-ing change due to MS is rarely a problem and, when acute episodes of hearing loss do occur, full recovery can be expected.

BLADDER AND BOWEL SYMPTOMS

Bladder Control: The most common symptoms of bladder involvement in MS are the need to urinate *often* (frequency) and the need to urinate *now* (urgency). If these symptoms are particularly troublesome, involuntary wetting (incontinence) can occur because of difficulty getting to the bathroom in time. Many people manage this by being aware of their symptoms and taking opportunities to urinate regularly. Markedly restricting fluid intake, which seems to be a logical method of dealing with the problem, is actually a bad idea; your kidneys and bladder need a continuous flow of fluids to excrete wastes and minimize the opportunity for infection.

If frequency and urgency are more serious problems and cannot be managed by simple measures, medications such as oxybutynin chloride (Ditropan), propantheline bromide (Pro-Banthine), tolterodine tartrate (Detrol), or flavoxate hydrochloride (Urispas) may control the problem. It is important to determine that urinary retention is not present before these medications are initiated. A number of problems with the bladder can occur in MS, each of which needs a specific approach to management. If simple measures and these medications are not sufficient to control the problem, a urologic assessment is needed to see if other approaches are required.

It is important to know that bladder problems are common in MS and that they can be managed with simple measures in most cases, but also that they can lead to serious complications if untreated. Urinary infection in men should always be explored further, and recurrent urinary tract infection in women also requires investigation. If burning or painful urination occurs, especially when the urine is cloudy and has a foul odor, you probably have a bladder infection and need to be in touch with your physician right away.

Bladder symptoms sometimes can be reduced by drinking about eight glasses (64 ounces total) of fluid daily, limiting citrus juices (orange, grapefruit, and tomato juices), and adding cranberry juice or cranberry tablets several times daily, which reduce infections.

Bowel Control: Bowel control problems (primarily constipation) are less common than bladder problems, and in most cases they also can be managed by simple methods. The first step is to maintain a regular bowel schedule. Try to have a bowel movement each day after breakfast because establishing a regular daily pattern avoids constipation and a tendency to irregular bowel movements as a result of inactivity. Each day take the time to sit and try at the same time—do not wait until you feel like going to the bathroom—to try to develop a regular reflex timing for bowel movements. Your diet should be high in fiber, including a serving of bran each day, and there should be adequate fruits and vegetables in your meals. Drinking enough fluid is also critical, as hard, dry stool is the most common cause of constipation.

Another factor in bowel health is exercise—this helps maintain good bowel function in everyone, but it is especially important when you have MS. Loss of bowel control is a more serious problem and can be managed by altering diet and some exercises, and in some cases medication will help. A consultation with a gastroenterologist may be needed if the bowel problems persist, especially if there is poor bowel control, because this problem can discourage a person from taking part in many social and family activities.

OTHER SYMPTOMS

Fatigue: People with MS may notice two patterns of fatigue. One is a feeling of tiredness and weakness that occurs with increasing exercise or other physical activity. For instance, walking may be fine at the onset, but your legs may become increasingly heavy and tired after walking a long distance, with some dragging of the feet. Strength is recovered and you can continue again after sitting down and resting for a brief time.

Another kind of fatigue is a general feeling of exhaustion, which can be more annoying and limiting. This can be mild or severe, intermittent or continuous. You may experience this type of fatigue quite suddenly during a normal day, which may come over you like a wave, making it difficult to continue with whatever you are doing.

More commonly, a general fatigue is present no matter how much or how little you do. It may be aggravated by overdoing activity or getting less sleep, but it may be present even if you do nothing and have had a good night's sleep. When we ask people with MS to list the symptoms that bother them the most, fatigue usually is at the top of the list; it also is the most common.

Most people learn to modify their day in ways that allow them to manage fatigue, such as taking brief rests or even occasional naps. Others say that they cannot do this because of the nature of their work or responsibilities, and they push through the fatigue without causing any problems. It simply makes you tired to overdo it when you have fatigue; it does not worsen your MS. The most common problem from overdoing things is to be more tired. It is common for people to say they can push through their work or task but that they pay for this effort with several days of increased fatigue. Some find their fatigue occurs at the same time each day, which may allow for some restructuring of activities in work or other schedules to manage the fatigue better.

Most people with MS say that the fatigue they experience feels abnormal, unlike the normal tiredness that everyone experiences. Most neurological diseases are not associated with this pattern of tiredness, although a number of other autoimmune diseases do exhibit unusual fatigue. Because it is so "different" and so common in MS, it is surprising that it was not recognized as a characteristic symptom of MS until recently. If you are experiencing fatigue, it is important to take a careful look at your typical day. You are subject to the same fatigue from overactivity as anyone else and the fatigue you are experiencing may not be due to MS.

Cognitive Impairment: People with MS, sometimes even those with a new diagnosis, may experience difficulty remembering things, finding the right words, or concentrating. These problems might reflect *cognitive impairment*—problems with thinking and memory that occur in about 50 to 60 percent of people with MS, which are generally unrelated to disease duration or seriousness of other symptoms. Fortunately, most people do not have extensive difficulty, and compensatory activities can be introduced, such as establishing regular routines (e.g., always putting the house keys in the same place), relying more on written information (such as written driving directions), and using a day calendar to track important activities. Formal testing can be done to identify any problems you are having so that a management plan can be tailored to your needs. If you are concerned about cognitive function, discuss this with your MS doctor, nurse, or mental health professional so that the issue can be addressed.

Tremor: Everyone has some tremor (to see the normal physiologic tremor, put a piece of paper on top of your outstretched hand). Multiple sclerosis may be accompanied by different types of tremor, ranging from annoying to fairly disabling. There are a variety of approaches to controlling them, some of which people learn on their own. For example, bracing the forearm against the side or on a hard surface reduces arm and hand tremor. Another variation is to have a method of immobilization that is used for some specific task, such as writing, but is removed when the task is completed. Physical and occupational therapists may use *patterning*, repeating movements to make them smoother and more automatic. Adding weights to the limb may reduce tremor, and adaptive equipment can be useful.

Medication is only partially effective, and some of the drugs tried in the past seemed to give only limited assistance and caused side effects. Perhaps the only drugs that may have a significant effect are beta blockers such as propranolol (Inderal). Mild sedatives and tranquilizers may help, but they probably are only worthwhile when you have some other need for a sedative, such as tension or anxiety, that aggravate tremor. There are studies showing that selective injections of onabotulinum toxin-A can improve marked tremor. Although this can weaken the muscles injected, this was found to be mild and resolved in a few weeks. Stereotactic brain surgery has been used in selected cases, but this is unusual and carries significant risk.

Vertigo: Vertigo is the sensation that many people call "dizziness," but since that term can mean different things, it is necessary to explain exactly what you feel. Vertigo has the sensation of movement, whether it seems that the room is moving or turning or that *you* seem to be moving. If it is severe, the room seems to be spinning, or you may feel like you are tipping or falling or that the floor is coming up to meet you. This sensation usually is due to a disturbance in the vestibular system of the middle ear or its connections within the brainstem and brain. In MS, the problem most often is in the nerve connections in the brainstem. It usually is transient, lasting hours or occasionally weeks; it is unusual for it to last much longer. If it persists, it can be treated by stimulating the vestibular system or by suppressing the vestibular reflexes with medication. If the onset of vertigo is acute and lasts for many days, it can be treated by intravenous steroids, but it usually resolves by itself. When vertigo is worsened by movement, as it often is, paradoxically the problem can be reduced by purposely stimulating the vertigo. Thus, positional exercises can be done using a simple method on a soft surface such as a bed. The vestibular system is stimulated by falling onto the bed to one side three times (the vertigo lessens each time), then to the other side, and then backward. There often is a position of comfort when a person has vertigo, with fewer symptoms when lying on one side and more symptoms when lying on the other side, and with the head supported at a certain angle. Sedatives are helpful, as is diazepam (Valium), which suppresses the vestibular reflex.

Vertigo can be mild, experienced as a slight swimming feeling in the head. Mild nausea and poor concentration often are associated with this. Again, positional exercises and an exercise program are more helpful than sitting still, which is the natural tendency.

Seizures: Seizures are not common in MS but occur in about 6 percent of patients. They usually are effectively treated with common anticonvulsants such as phenytoin (Dilantin) or carbamazepine (Tegretol). An unusual type of "seizure" is a localized spasm that is more like a major muscle spasm than an epileptic seizure and often occurs on one side of the body. Such spasms also respond to medication such as carbamazepine.

Facial Weakness: Facial weakness can occur suddenly in MS, although it is uncommon. When it does happen, especially early in the course of the disease, it may resemble Bell's palsy, a benign form of acute facial palsy that often follows a viral infection. Both Bell's palsy and the facial weakness of MS respond to steroids. In MS, no treatment may be needed if the weakness is mild or is already rapidly improving on its own.

Summary

MS brings with it many uncertainties about the future. However, what is certain is that MS is treatable, with many new therapies on the horizon. You have every reason to be optimistic about your future and the promise of better treatments to come. Be sure you have the best health care team for your needs, then work closely with them, and your MS society, to maintain the highest possible quality of life.

CHAPTER 5

Unconventional Medicines and Multiple Sclerosis

People who are recently diagnosed with MS often look to unconventional and alternative medicines in the hopes of finding something that might be helpful for their disease or their symptoms. There are hundreds of these therapies available from health food stores, on-line, or from therapists. How can you find information that is reliable about so many products and procedures, and evidence about whether a product or therapy is effective and safe? There is great variability in the quantity and quality of information about these therapies, sometimes coming only from the person selling the therapy, but in others there may be clinical studies allowing you to judge the claims. Also, some are cheap and others expensive. Some are safe and others have known serious side effects and complications. Consequently, it is especially important to be knowledgeable and cautious in this area.

This chapter provides background information about unconventional medicine, strategies for evaluating unconventional therapies, and MS-specific information about unconventional therapies that are popular or are particularly relevant to MS.

Definitions

Unconventional medicine is a term that is surprisingly difficult to define. Part of the difficulty is that many different terms are used. In addition to *unconventional medicine*, other frequently used terms include *alternative medicine, complementary medicine,* and *integrative medicine.* These are often referred to as CAM, for complementary and alternative medicine, referring to treatments that are not part of standard medical care. One of the more commonly used terms is *unconventional medicine.* This is sometimes defined as therapies that are not typically taught in medical schools or generally available as standard care in hospitals. However, this definition is awkward because it states what unconventional medicine *is not,* as opposed to what it *is.* Also, this definition is a "moving target" because it depends on the medical traditions of the country in which it is used, and in some countries, including the United States, many medical schools now offer courses in unconventional medicine. Also, if something unconventional can be shown to be effective it may then become standard care.

There are many other definitions of unconventional medicine. One definition that is more precise, but also more complex, is provided by the National Institutes of Health (NIH). There is a branch of the NIH that provides information and research on CAM called the National Center for Complementary and Alternative Medicine.

In the NIH definition, unconventional medicine is subdivided into categories. These categories, with representative examples, include:

- Biologically based therapies: Dietary supplements, diets, bee venom therapy
- Mind-body therapies: Guided imagery, hypnosis, meditation
- Alternative medical systems: Traditional Chinese medicine, ayurveda, homeopathy

- Manipulative and body-based therapies: Chiropractic, reflexology, massage
- Energy therapies: Therapeutic touch, magnets

Other terms refer to the way in which the therapies are used. Unconventional therapies that are used instead of conventional medicine are known as *alternative medicine*, while unconventional therapies that are used in conjunction with conventional medicine are called *complementary medicine.* An even broader term, *integrative medicine*, refers to the combined use of conventional and unconventional medicine.

There have been many studies of the use of CAM in the general population and in people with MS. In studies in several countries, it has been found that about one half to three fourths of people with MS use some form of unconventional medicine, usually in conjunction with therapies recommended by their physicians. In other words, the unconventional medicine is used as *complementary medicine.*

Evidence for the Safety and Effectiveness of Therapies

Before using an alternative therapy it is important to get information on what evidence there is for its effectiveness and also its risks. Often the claims of benefit and safety commonly come from personal stories or from people selling the remedy, but without any published clinical trials or convincing scientific evidence.

Statements that things are "natural" are insufficient to guarantee either benefit or freedom from side effects. That a therapy has been around a long time, even centuries, is also not assurance of benefit. Bleeding was used a therapy for thousands of years until some of the earliest clinical trials showed it was not helpful and even harmful in some patients. Different types of evidence may be available to determine the safety and effectiveness of unconventional as well as conventional therapies. Information about a therapy may be based on personal stories, theoretical arguments, experimental studies, or clinical trials of people with MS. When reviewing information about a therapy, it is important to determine the strength of available evidence. Some CAM literature does not distinguish between the various levels of evidence and may make very strong recommendations on the basis of weak evidence.

Ideally, for any therapy, whether conventional or unconventional, there should be scientific evidence for the claimed benefits, and clear evidence for the risks.

People with MS who are interested in CAM should use a careful and thoughtful approach that is similar to that used for conventional therapies for which the evidence is limited. It is important to obtain unbiased MS-relevant information, evaluate the safety and effectiveness of the therapy, and discuss the therapy with your physician or other conventional health care provider. If a therapy is pursued, there should be a plan for monitoring for an expected response. If that response does not occur, the therapy should be discontinued and other approaches considered. It is important to use caution, realize that the safety and effectiveness information about most CAM therapies is limited, and recognize that there is a certain degree of risk in pursuing any CAM therapy.

Using Complementary and Alternative Medicine

It can be reasonable to use CAM in some circumstances, such as taking a treatment that seems safe for mild fatigue or mild muscle stiffness, or for symptoms for which conventional medicine has no effective therapies or only partially effective therapies. On the other hand, a serious disease such as MS should not be treated initially or exclusively with CAM therapies when there are effective therapies supported by clinical trial evidence of safety and benefit.

Some CAM books make erroneous claims about MS, some of which are potentially dangerous. One frequent misunderstanding is that because MS is an immune disease, it should be treated by stimulating the immune system with dietary supplements. This is incorrect. MS is an immune disease, but it is characterized by *excessive and abnormal* immune system activity. As a result, agents that have been proven to be effective in MS generally *decrease or modulate* the immune system activity.

Features of some CAM therapies that should raise concerns:

- "Secret ingredients," or little objective information about safety or effectiveness
- Extremely strong claims about effectiveness, such as claims that a single therapy is effective for many different conditions
- Use of "testimonials" in which individuals make strong claims about effectiveness

There are common misconceptions about dietary supplements, which include vitamins, minerals, and herbs. Some supplements are claimed to have therapeutic effects and no side effects, which is not true. Supplements, especially herbs, are similar to medications and contain chemicals that may produce beneficial effects but may also cause side effects. Also, it is sometimes claimed that "more is better," especially with vitamins and minerals, which can be not only incorrect but dangerous. Finally, it is sometimes stated that "natural" compounds are safe and beneficial, but some can be toxic, especially if taken in high doses, and many can have harmful interactions when taken with other medications.

Unconventional Therapies Relevant to MS

For some individuals, the thoughtful use of CAM therapies, especially in combination with conventional medicine, may allow for an individualized treatment plan and provide hope, control, and a sense of empowerment. The remainder of this chapter provides MS-relevant information about CAM therapies that have been specifically studied in MS, are used commonly in the general population or by people with MS, or raise specific safety concerns.

Acupuncture and Traditional Chinese Medicine

Acupuncture is one component of traditional Chinese medicine (TCM). Other components include traditional Chinese herbs, nutrition, exercise, stress reduction, and massage. TCM is based on a theory of body function that is very different from that of Western medicine. Specifically, it is believed that energy, or *qi*, flows through fourteen major pathways, or *meridians*, on the body. There is also a balance of opposites, which are known as *yin* and *yang*. According to TCM, disease occurs when there is disturbance or disharmony of energy. With acupuncture, thin, metallic needles are inserted in specific points on the meridians. It is believed that the insertion of acupuncture needles alters the flow of energy in such a way that it produces therapeutic effects.

There is limited information about *acupuncture* in people with MS. There have been a number of small and poorly designed trials to assess acupuncture in the treatment of MS but these have not been definitive enough to indicate effectiveness and acupuncture is not recommended in the treatment of MS. In fact, the theory of acupuncture is that it might stimulate the immune system, and there have been suggestions that it may worsen MS. There is better evidence for benefit of acupuncture in pain, and it may have a place if the MS patient is seeking relief of pain rather than treatment of the MS. Acupuncture is usually well tolerated, especially when it is done by a well-trained acupuncturist. Sterile needles should be used to avoid infections, including hepatitis and AIDS. Acupuncture is moderately expensive, especially as it often involves repeated treatments. When done by a well-trained therapist it is low risk.

The safety of *Chinese herbal medicine* has not been well characterized, especially in people with MS. There is a theoretical risk of worsening MS with immune-stimulating herbs, which include Asian ginseng, astragalus, and maitake and reishi mushrooms. In addition, one herb that mildly suppresses the immune system, thunder god vine (*Tripterygium wilfordii*), may produce serious side effects, including death. Chinese herbal medicine is a low-to-medium cost therapy, but with some risks and uncertain benefit.

Marijuana (Cannabis)

For years, it has been claimed that marijuana, also known as *cannabis*, is an effective treatment for MS. Marijuana, which is still illegal in many countries, contains compounds known as cannabinoids. These compounds, which include tetrahydrocannabinol (THC), produce specific biochemical effects in the body. Marijuana may be smoked or ingested. There are prescription medications that contain cannabinoids. In the United States, THC is available as dronabinol (Marinol). In Europe, Canada, and Australia, a synthetic form of THC is available as nabilone (Cesamet). An oral spray form of cannabis (Sativex) is approved in Canada for treating MS pain.

Cannabinoids exert several biological effects that, on a theoretical basis, could be therapeutic for MS. First, they bind to proteins in the central nervous system that suppress excessive nerve cell activity. This could result in a decrease in pain and muscle stiffness (spasticity). Also, cannabinoids bind to another type of protein on immune cells and mildly suppress the immune system. It is possible that cannabinoids could be beneficial in the course of MS but this has not been proven in clinical trials. It has some benefit in the treatment of pain and spasticity in MS.

There are mixed results in studies. In several surveys of people with MS who have smoked marijuana, symptoms commonly reported to be improved include pain, spasticity, depression, and anxiety. Importantly, surveys such as this are not rigorous enough to provide definitive evidence for effectiveness. Actual clinical studies of the effects of smoked or oral marijuana on MS symptoms are of variable quality.

Significant risks are associated with smoking marijuana, including nausea, vomiting, sedation, increased risk of seizures, and poor pregnancy outcomes. Driving may be impaired for up to 8 hours after smoking marijuana. High doses of marijuana may impair heart function, decrease reaction time, and produce coordination and visual difficulties. Chronic marijuana use may cause heart attacks, impair lung function, cause dependence and apathy, and increase the risk of cancer of the lung, head, and neck. An apathy syndrome develops in some chronic users. There is evidence that it may worsen schizophrenia and depression. Many patients do not like this as a form of therapy as it makes them feel "stoned" and they wanted pain relief, not to feel these other effects. Needless to say, there are legal problems if marijuana is used where the laws prohibit its use. It is legally available to MS patients for pain and spasticity in Canada, and steps toward legalization of marijuana are being taken, as in many U.S. states. Smoked marijuana and prescription medications containing cannabinoids are of low-moderate cost. Marijuana, where it is legal, has been used for some symptom relief of pain and spasticity, and may have some benefit for MS. The benefit is still unclear and under study.

Chiropractic Medicine

Chiropractic medicine is one of the most popular forms of CAM in the United States, with over 60,000 practitioners. Chiropractic medicine is based on the concept that the nervous system plays a critical role in health and that many diseases are caused by abnormal pressure of bones on the nerves in the spine. There are within chiropractic two groups—those who adhere to the original concepts and those who add newer ideas and other approaches to their practice.

Chiropractors believe that misalignments of the bones of the spine cause abnormal pressure on the nerves that travel from the spinal cord to the muscles and organs of the body that results in impaired muscle and organ function. Spinal manipulation techniques, known as "adjustments," are thought to normalize bone positions and restore normal function.

There are no well-designed studies that document that spinal manipulation or other chiropractic methods can alter the disease course in MS. Isolated clinical reports have described improvement in some MS symptoms with chiropractic treatment, but there are no systematic clinical studies of chiropractic treatment for MS symptoms.

Chiropractic treatment is generally well tolerated, but complications of manipulation can occur, and some are serious. One of the more common adverse effects is aching muscles, which may be present for one to two days after manipulation. A rare, but serious, complication associated with neck manipulation is stroke when arteries in the neck are damaged. Very rarely, low back manipulation may cause compression of the nerves of the lower spine (cauda equine syndrome). Pregnant women, people taking anticoagulant medications, and people with spinal bone fractures, spine trauma, significant disc herniations, bone cancer or infection, severe osteoporosis, and severe arthritis should avoid chiropractic therapy. Importantly, since chiropractors are not as well trained in diagnosis as physicians, people with serious diseases or conditions should be evaluated and treated by a physician and should not substitute chiropractic medicine for conventional medicine. Chiropractic therapy is of moderate cost but can be higher if a long course of therapy is carried out.

Cooling Therapy

Cooling therapy is a form of CAM that is unique to MS. It has been known for years that changes in body temperature may significantly affect MS symptoms. Specifically, small increases in body temperature (32.9°F, 0.5°C) may worsen symptoms, while small decreases may improve symptoms. Consequently, various cooling methods have been developed. These methods range from simple techniques, such as drinking cold liquids and staying in air-conditioned areas, to complex methods, such as using specially designed cooling suits. Cooling suits may be *passive* or *active*. Passive garments use ice packs for cooling; active garments use circulating coolants.

Beneficial effects of cooling garments have been noted in several clinical studies. Unfortunately, some of these reports are preliminary and most of the studies have been small and not rigorously conducted. Among these studies, improvement in fatigue is frequently seen. Other symptoms showing transient improvement include leg weakness, spasticity, difficulty walking, bladder dysfunction, sexual difficulties, visual changes, speech difficulties, cognitive difficulties, and incoordination. The results of the most rigorous cooling study in MS showed by objective measures that cooling was associated with mildly improved walking and visual function. By subjective measures, cooling improved fatigue, strength, and cognition. Cooling garments may be especially well suited for those who are most heat sensitive.

The use of cooling garments is usually well tolerated. Some people feel uncomfortable when cooling begins, and some cooling suits are cumbersome, particularly the active circulating suits that require attachment to a motor to keep a coolant circulating. Some people with MS have a paradoxical sensitivity to cold, in which case cooling may actually *worsen* symptoms. This is by a different mechanism, as cooling can further tighten the muscles that are stiff and spastic.

Costs of cooling are dependent on the method used. Simple techniques are of low cost. Passive cooling garments are of moderate cost. Active cooling devices are expensive.

Dental Amalgam Removal

Removal of dental amalgam has been proposed as a treatment method for MS. For more than 150 years, cavities have been filled with dental amalgam, which is composed of mercury as well as silver, copper, tin, and zinc. Amalgam is currently used in about 80 to 90 percent of tooth restorations.

Although some have argued without convincing evidence that the mercury in dental amalgam might be related to the cause of MS on the grounds that if some mercury were absorbed it could damage the nervous system or its presence could generate electrical activity. There is no convincing evidence that mercury or the presence of dental amalgam has anything to do with causing MS, so there is no reason to remove the dental fillings. Paradoxically, removal of mercury fillings may increase the blood levels of mercury.

Studies of trace metals in MS using a Slow Poke Atomic Reactor showed no abnormal levels in MS patients and no difference from a normal control group. Dental amalgam removal as a treatment for

MS is not supported by multiple professional organizations, including the National Multiple Sclerosis Society of the United States. Removal of dental fillings is moderately expensive but not recommended.

Dietary Supplements

A wide range of compounds is included in the category of dietary supplements. Vitamins, minerals, and herbs are commonly used supplements. Other diverse compounds, including amino acids, hormones, and enzymes, are also classified as dietary supplements. In this section, dietary supplements that are popular or are relevant to MS are addressed.

Antioxidants

Free radicals are chemicals that may injure cells in the body through a process known as *oxidative damage*. Antioxidants are compounds that can decrease oxidative damage. Commonly used antioxidants include selenium and vitamins A, C, and E. Other compounds in the antioxidant category include alpha-lipoic acid, inosine, uric acid, coenzyme Q10 (CoQ10), grape seed extract, pycnogenol, and oligomeric proanthocyanidins (OPCs). Antioxidants are sometimes specifically marketed as a treatment for MS.

There are two major reasons that antioxidants could be considered in MS. First, it could be theorized that free radicals may be involved in the pathology of MS by damaging the myelin around nerves if free radicals were released by immune cells. Also, the nerve fibers themselves, the axons, are damaged in MS through a degenerative process that may involve free radicals. Indeed, some studies indicate that oxidative damage is increased in experimental allergic encephalomyelitis (EAE), the animal model of MS, and in tissue from people with MS.

Specific studies of antioxidants in MS are very limited. Studies in EAE indicate that antioxidants may decrease disease severity. Recent studies have shown that alpha-lipoic acid and uric acid are effective in mice with EAE. Clinical studies in people with MS are currently being conducted with alpha-lipoic acid and inosine, a compound that is converted to uric acid.

Since many antioxidant compounds activate immune cells that are already excessively active in MS, further stimulation by antioxidants could potentially worsen the disease. Whether this occurs and is clinically important in MS has not been investigated and remains a theoretical risk.

The safety of many dietary supplements, including antioxidants, has not been determined in women who are pregnant or breastfeeding. Supplementation with antioxidants is a low-cost therapy.

Cranberry and Other Supplements Used for Urinary Tract Infections

People with MS are prone to bladder difficulties, including urinary tract infections (UTIs). There is a long-held belief that cranberry juice and related products might prevent recurrent infections but recent studies in susceptible populations such as nursing home residents did not show any benefit over a placebo. The ideal clinical trial with cranberry has not been done in MS patients but there is little reason to believe it would be more beneficial in MS patients. There is also little evidence for two other UTI-related dietary supplements, vitamin C and bearberry.

Cranberry is inexpensive and generally well tolerated. Cranberry tablets are less expensive than juice. Cranberry may interfere with blood-thinning medications, such as warfarin (Coumadin). Long-term use of high doses may increase the risk of kidney stones and may cause gastrointestinal discomfort, loose stools, and nausea. There is insufficient information about the safety of cranberry in women who are pregnant or breastfeeding.

Echinacea and Other "Immune-Stimulating" Supplements

Echinacea and several other dietary supplements are known to activate the immune system, leading some therapists to suggest that MS patients should take echinacea and other dietary supplement.

This is a potentially dangerous concept because MS is character-ized by increased immune activity and compounds that stimulate the immune system could worsen the disease. However, many dietary supplements and herbals said to stimulate the immune system actu-ally do not have any effect on the immune mechanisms so probably do not help or worsen MS.

The immune system effects of some dietary supplements have undergone limited investigation in test-tube or animal experiments. These studies have investigated components of the immune sys-tem that are excessively active in MS. Activation of these cells has been produced by echinacea and several other dietary supplements, including:

- Herbs: Alfalfa, Asian ginseng, astragalus, cat's claw, garlic, maitake mushroom, mistletoe, shiitake mushroom, Siberian ginseng, stinging nettle
- Vitamins and minerals: Antioxidant vitamins and minerals (see the preceding section on "Antioxidants"), zinc
- Melatonin

Based on scientific evidence, these compounds pose theoretical risks to people with MS.

Ginkgo Biloba

Ginkgo biloba usually refers to the extract that is derived from the leaf of the *Ginkgo biloba* tree. Among herbs, ginkgo is one of the most extensively studied and one of the most popular. There are sev-eral effects of ginkgo that might suggest a use in MS. Ginkgo has anti-inflammatory and antioxidant effects. Also ginkgo was thought to improve cognitive function in people with Alzheimer's disease, although clinical trials have not borne this out.

Ginkgo has undergone limited investigation in MS. Ginkgo and related compounds decreased disease severity in some, but not all, studies in the animal model of MS.

Although a small study suggested it might be helpful in reducing MS attacks, a larger and more rigorously conducted trial failed to show any benefit. Thus, it does not appear to be effective for MS attacks. There are no convincing studies of ginkgo for other benefits in MS such as reducing the course of the disease or improving cognitive function, and there is growing concern about the side effects and dangers of ginkgo.

Ginkgo is usually well tolerated in low doses. It may have a blood-thinning effect and thus should be avoided in people who have bleeding disorders, or who take antiplatelet or anticoagulant medication, or are undergoing surgery. It can provoke seizures and should be used with caution by those with seizure disorders. It may also cause dizziness, rashes, headache, and gastrointestinal complaints, including nausea, vomiting, diarrhea, and flatulence. The safety of ginkgo in women who are pregnant or breastfeeding is not known. Most medicinal ginkgo is made from the leaf; in some counties the seeds are used, and these are much more dangerous. Ginkgo is inexpensive.

St. John's Wort

St. John's wort is not a treatment for MS but is sometimes used by patients who are suffering from symptoms of depression, and depression is a relatively common symptom in patients who have MS. It is so named because it blooms around the time of the feast day of St. John the Baptist (June 24). The red pigments in its buds and flowers are associated with the blood of St. John the Baptist.

Some small studies suggested that St. John's wort had benefit in milder depression, but there was no greater effect than a placebo in a large study. There is no evidence that St. John's wort is effective for treating severe depression. It is unclear how the effectiveness of St. John's wort compares to that of the newer antidepressants known as selective serotonin reuptake inhibitors (SSRIs), such as fluoxetine (Prozac), paroxetine (Paxil), and sertraline (Zoloft).

Although St. John's wort is usually well tolerated, there are several important factors related to its use. People who are concerned they may have depression should not attempt to diagnose and treat this condition on their own. St. John's wort may worsen MS fatigue or increase the sedating effects of some medications. St. John's wort may cause a sensitivity of the skin and nerves to sunlight ("photo-sensitivity"), especially in those who are fair skinned. It should be avoided by women who are pregnant or breastfeeding because of possible side effects. Finally, St. John's wort may alter the levels of multiple drugs, including anticonvulsants, antidepressants, heart medications, blood-thinning medications, and oral contraceptives. St. John's wort is inexpensive.

Valerian

People with MS are prone to sleep disorders. Valerian, an herb that has been used for more than 1,000 years, may be helpful for treating insomnia. The mechanism by which valerian might produce its actions is unclear.

Several clinical studies of variable reliability have suggested that valerian is effective for treating insomnia. Valerian is also sometimes claimed to be effective for depression and muscle stiffness (spasticity). However, due to limited clinical studies, its effects on these conditions are not known. A review of nine studies of valerian on sleep by the National Center for Complementary and Alternative Medicine at the National Institutes of Health concluded that the results, some negative and some positive, were too variable to be conclusive about whether valerian was effective in the treatment of sleep disorders.

Valerian is generally safe. It may cause sedation, which may worsen MS fatigue or increase the sedating effects of some medications. The safety of long-term use and use during pregnancy or breastfeeding has not been established. Valerian is inexpensive.

Vitamin B_{12} (Cobalamin, Cyanocobalamin)

Supplements of vitamin B_{12}, also known as cobalamin or cyanocobalamin, are sometimes claimed to be effective therapies for MS.

Vitamin B_{12} is essential for maintaining normal nervous system functioning. Almost all people get enough vitamin B_{12} from their normal diet and need no additional supplements. Exceptions are people with pernicious anemia, who cannot absorb B_{12}, and rarely strict vegans whose diet is so limited that they do not get enough natural B_{12} in their diet. People with vitamin B_{12} deficiency, like some people with MS, have injury to the optic nerves and the spinal cord. For these and other reasons, it is sometimes concluded that vitamin B_{12} supplements could be effective MS therapies but there is no convincing supportive evidence.

The mechanism by which nervous system injury occurs in MS is different from that associated with vitamin B_{12} deficiency. In addition, most people with MS have normal vitamin B_{12} levels. For people who have normal vitamin B_{12} levels, there is no evidence that vitamin B_{12} supplements provide any significant beneficial effects.

Vitamin B_{12} supplements are usually well tolerated. It can be taken by oral tablets or wafers, but in pernicious anemia must be taken by injection. Rarely, vitamin B_{12} may cause diarrhea, rashes, and itching. Vitamin B_{12} is inexpensive.

Vitamin D and Calcium

There is a lot of research on the possible role of vitamin D in the potential cause, treatment, and prevention of MS. A large conference on vitamin D and MS evaluated the current evidence and the studies necessary to answer many questions.

Vitamin D and calcium have multiple actions in the body, including an important role in maintaining bone density. Vitamin D and calcium are relevant to people with MS because people with MS are at risk for developing osteoporosis and a less severe form of decreased bone density known as osteopenia. In addition, vitamin D and calcium are involved in the immune system function in a way that could be therapeutic for people with MS (see Chapter 4).

A possible therapeutic effect for vitamin D in MS is suggested by several studies. In the animal model resembling MS, disease severity is worsened by vitamin D deficiency and improved by vitamin D supplementation. A recent observation that will have implications for therapy trials is that the protective effects of vitamin D in the animal model of MS seemed to be in the females but not the males, suggesting that estrogen may be essential to the protective effect.

Epidemiologic studies indicate that the use of vitamin D supplements is associated with a decreased risk of developing MS, and those with low blood levels of vitamin D are at greater risk of MS than those with higher levels. This was found in a large British nurses health study and also in a study of U.S. veterans, and there are more recent supportive studies.

Unfortunately, there is very limited clinical trial information about vitamin D as a treatment of MS, although such studies are currently being designed and a few are already underway. There are short-term studies suggesting some reduction in relapses and in fewer new lesions on the MRI with vitamin D therapy. Although vitamin D research is taking many interesting directions, a large randomized clinical trial is difficult to arrange as so many people are now taking vitamin D, which is so easily available. It will be difficult to keep strict control over a large population of patients in the two groups, treatment and placebo, over a number of years.

No one knows what the dose should be, but larger and larger doses are being tried, often in the 2,000 to 5,000 IU range. A study of tolerance to high dosage showed that MS patients could tolerate a course of 40,000 IU, then lowering the dosage to 10,000 IU daily, without much difficulty. The concern would be with prolonged therapy as we do not know the overall risks of long-term treatment with high doses in MS populations.

In reasonable doses, vitamin D and calcium are usually well tolerated. Calcium may interfere with the absorption of some medications (antibiotics, thyroid medication, osteoporosis medication) and minerals (iron, magnesium, zinc). In high doses, vitamin D and calcium may cause multiple side effects. Vitamin D and calcium are inexpensive and available without a prescription.

Diets

Many diets have been proposed as effective MS therapies. For many of these diets, there is no clear underlying rationale or clinical evidence to support their use in MS. Diets for MS that are not supported by a strong rationale or clinical data include allergen-free diets, gluten-free diets, pectin-restricted diets, fructose-restricted diets, severely sugar-restricted diets, and diets that reduce or eliminate processed foods.

On the basis of scientific, epidemiologic, animal model, and clinical trial studies, there is suggestive evidence that diets that are low in saturated fats and high in polyunsaturated fatty acids (PUFAs) may have a therapeutic effect in MS. PUFAs include omega-3 and omega-6 fatty acids. Omega-6 fatty acids include compounds known as linoleic acid and gamma-linolenic acid. Examples of omega-3 fatty acids include eicosapentaenoic acid (EPA), docosahexaenoic acid (DHA), and alpha-linolenic acid (ALA). The first PUFA-enriched diet that was extensively studied in MS was the Swank diet. Subsequently, several MS clinical studies evaluated the effects of supplementation with omega-6 and omega-3 fatty acids.

The Swank Diet

In the 1940s, Dr. Roy Swank developed a dietary approach to MS that was low in saturated fat. With this diet, saturated fat intake is decreased to 15 grams (g) or less daily, high-fat dairy products are excluded, frequent fish meals are recommended, and 10 to 15 g of fluid vegetable oil and 5 g of cod liver oil are added to the daily diet.

Dr. Swank reported on his group of treated patients over many decades, suggesting their rate of MS attacks was decreased by 70 percent relative to the attack rate prior to entering the study. Unfortunately, there was no control group to compare these results, and no indication of how those who dropped out of the study fared, so it is difficult to know if these patients would have done the same without the dietary change. Also, over time, the number of attacks of MS is expected to come down. However he did note that compared to untreated MS patients in the literature, his patients had less frequent attacks, less progression of neurological disability, and decreased mortality. These beneficial effects were greatest in those who adhered strictly to the diet and those who were mildly affected or were early in the course of the disease. Although these findings were encouraging, it needed to be confirmed with a blinded randomized clinical trial, as his patients were not selected randomly, there was no placebo group, and the patients and the physician were not "blinded" as to who was on treatment versus on placebo, with follow-up of all patients, including those who drop out of the study. Due to these and other shortcomings, this study is not rigorous enough to provide definitive conclusions about the effectiveness of this dietary approach. It is recognized that a long-term, blinded dietary study with a control diet group is very difficult to perform. In the 1980 three studies were done and two suggested some benefit on reducing attacks and an analysis of all three together suggested some benefit on attacks and disability in the mildest cases of MS. A subsequent rigorous trial did not show a statistically significant benefit, but a trend toward benefit in disability progression.

This Swank diet is usually well tolerated. Long-term adherence to the diet may not be possible because the recommended food is not appealing. Due to the decreased meat intake in the Swank diet, people who use this dietary approach should be certain that their protein intake is adequate. Although cod liver oil, one component of this diet, is generally safe, it may rarely cause adverse effects. Cod liver oil may have a blood-thinning effect and should be used with caution by those who take aspirin or anticoagulant medication, are undergoing surgery, or have bleeding disorders. Diabetics should also use cod liver oil with caution. Finally, cod liver oil contains relatively high concentrations of vitamin A, which may be toxic in doses greater than 10,000 IU. The Swank diet is inexpensive.

Supplementation with Omega-6 Fatty Acids

Supplementation with omega-6 fatty acids is an approach that increases the intake of polyunsaturated fatty acids (PUFAs). Most studies of omega-6 fatty acid supplementation have used sunflower seed oil or evening primrose oil. Other dietary supplements that contain omega-6 fatty acids include flaxseed oil, borage seed oil, black currant seed oil, and spirulina (blue-green algae).

As noted for the Swank diet, epidemiologic studies indicate that a high intake of PUFAs may be associated with a lower risk of developing MS. There are other findings that support the use of a diet enriched in omega-6 fatty acids. Some, but not all, studies have shown that the blood levels of PUFAs are decreased in people with MS. In addition, scientific studies show that in the body PUFAs are converted to compounds that have anti-inflammatory effects and immune system–modulating effects that, on a theoretical basis, could be therapeutic for MS.

In the animal model of MS, disease severity is worsened by deficiencies in omega-6 fatty acids and lessened by supplementation with omega-6 fatty acids. In people with relapsing-remitting MS, three placebo-controlled clinical trials have evaluated supplementation with omega-6 fatty acids as part of the low PUFA diet already mentioned. As mentioned an analysis of these diet-supplement studies showed a benefit over the placebo groups in the milder groups of MS, but no effect in those with greater disability. In studies of people with progressive MS, omega-6 fatty acid supplementation has not been effective. Evening primrose oil, a dietary supplement that contains an omega-6 fatty acid known as gamma-linolenic acid has not produced therapeutic effects in people with relapsing-remitting or progressive disease.

Supplementation with omega-6 fatty acids is usually well tolerated. The safety of long-term supplementation with omega-6 fatty acids has not been well studied. A concern has been raised that linoleic acid supplementation may increase the risk of some forms of cancer, but this has not been proven. Since supplementation with PUFAs may cause vitamin E deficiency, supplementation with vitamin E may be necessary. Evening primrose oil, and perhaps other gamma–linolenic acid–containing supplements (black currant seed oil, borage seed oil, spirulina), may rarely provoke seizures. Also, gamma–linolenic acid–containing supplements may have blood-thinning effects. Omega-6 fatty acid supplements may increase triglyceride levels and thus should be used with caution by people with elevated triglycerides. One specific supplement, borage seed oil, may contain liver toxins. The safety of black currant seed oil has not been well studied. Spirulina products may contain heavy metals, bacteria, and other contaminants. The safety of omega-6 fatty acid supplementation in women who are pregnant or breastfeeding is not known. Supplementation with omega-6 fatty acids is inexpensive.

Supplementation with Omega-3 Fatty Acids

This approach increases the intake of omega-3 fatty acids, which include eicosapentaenoic acid (EPA), docosahexaenoic acid (DHA), and alpha-linolenic acid (ALA). EPA and DHA are present in relatively high levels in fish, especially fatty fish such as salmon, Atlantic herring, Atlantic mackerel, bluefin tuna, and sardines. Dietary supplements containing EPA and DHA include fish oil and cod liver oil. Rich sources of ALA include flaxseed oil, canola oil, and walnut oil.

The rationale for this approach is similar to that outlined for the Swank diet and supplementation with omega-6 fatty acids. In addition, immunologic studies indicate that, among the polyunsaturated fatty acids (PUFAs), the omega-3 fatty acids exert the most potent anti-inflammatory and immune-modulating effects. Also, omega-3 fatty acids appear to be important in forming and maintaining myelin, a part of the nervous system that is injured in MS.

Studies of omega-3 fatty acid supplementation in the animal model of MS are limited and conflicting. The most rigorous clinical study of this approach was a placebo-controlled trial of fish oil in people with relapsing-remitting MS. There was a trend for the treated group to show less disease progression, fewer attacks, and decreased attack duration, but these findings were minimal and not statistically significant. Therapeutic effects were noted in two uncontrolled studies, one with cod liver oil, calcium, and magnesium, and the other with fish oil, other dietary supplements, and dietary advice. A small study evaluated omega-3 fatty acid supplementation in combination with interferons or glatiramer acetate. People were treated with their MS medications along with either fish oil plus a very low-fat diet, or with olive oil and a low-fat diet. There was a trend for improved physical and emotional functioning in those taking fish oil. Both dietary interventions were associated with a decrease in relapse rate.

Fish oils are certified as generally safe for use by the U.S. Food and Drug Administration. The long-term safety of other omega-3 fatty acid supplements is not known. Increased dietary intake of ALA may increase the risk of prostate cancer. Although fish oil supplements generally do not have a significant amount of mercury, some fish, such as shark, swordfish, and king mackerel, do contain relatively high mercury levels. Fish and flaxseed oil may have a blood-thinning effect. Fish oil may impair lung function in those who are aspirin sensitive. High doses of fish oil may increase blood sugar levels in diabetics. High doses of flaxseed oil may produce cyanide toxicity. There are potential side effects that are specifically associated with cod liver oil (see the discussion of the Swank diet). For women who are pregnant or breastfeeding, the safety of omega-3 fatty acid supplements, including fish oil, is not known. Supplementation with omega-3 fatty acids is inexpensive.

Other Types of Therapy

Feldenkrais

Feldenkrais, a type of bodywork, teaches comfortable and efficient body movements. It is claimed to improve multiple symptoms and to provide therapeutic effects for people with MS. The retraining of movements with Feldenkrais is believed to increase the efficiency and comfort of body movements. This is claimed to improve walking stability, increase strength and coordination, and decrease stress.

Feldenkrais has undergone very limited investigation in MS and other conditions. In one small study, twenty people with MS were treated for eight weeks with either Feldenkrais or sham sessions. The treated group had significantly decreased stress and a trend for decreased anxiety relative to the sham group. This study was not rigorous enough to be conclusive.

Feldenkrais is generally safe and of low-moderate cost.

Guided Imagery and Relaxation

Guided imagery, also known as *imagery* or *visualization*, is a relaxation method, often used in combination with other relaxation methods, such as progressive muscle relaxation. It is claimed to be effective for treating a variety of symptoms including anxiety, depression, and pain. In guided imagery, an individual creates mental images that have specific effects on the body and mind.

In one published study of thirty-three people with MS, it was found that anxiety was decreased, but these methods had no effect on depression or other MS symptoms. Guided imagery and relaxation are usually well tolerated. Relaxation may cause or worsen muscle stiffness. Imagery may cause fear of losing control, anxiety, and disturbing thoughts, and so people with psychiatric conditions should use it with caution. Guided imagery is inexpensive.

Hyperbaric Oxygen

Hyperbaric oxygen (HBO) treatment is a form of oxygen therapy in which a person breathes oxygen under increased pressure in a specially designed pressure chamber. The oxygen content of the blood increases with the use of HBO that results in an increased amount of oxygen in different body tissues. HBO is an accepted treatment for a limited number of specific medical conditions, including carbon monoxide poisoning, burns, severe infections, gas gangrene, and decompression sickness (due to deep-sea diving). Unfortunately, there is no accepted evidence to support the use of HBO in MS. Although there was an initial trial that suggested some benefit, this has not been borne out in subsequent trials. Many clinical trials were conducted and found that HBO did not produce beneficial effects in people with MS. Two large independent reviews of all studies of HBO in MS concluded there is no therapeutic effect of HBO in people with MS and that HBO should not be used to treat MS. In addition, the Cochrane Collaboration, which conducts reviews of clinical trials, concluded that on the basis of current evidence further studies of HBO in MS are not justified. Despite the negative conclusions, the initial enthusiasm for HBO therapy resulted in numerous pressure chambers being placed in clinics, and this procedure is still available.

HBO is usually well tolerated. Reversible, mild visual symptoms may occur. Rarely, HBO may cause serious side effects, including seizures, collapsed lungs, pressure injury to the ear, and cataracts. HBO is expensive.

Magnetic Field Therapy (Electromagnetic Therapy)

There are two main forms of this therapy: static, permanent magnets and pulsed electromagnetic fields. Static magnetic therapy involves the use of magnetized devices such as bracelets, belts, and mattress pads. Although these devices are widely available and sold for many different conditions there is no evidence or accepted rationale for their use.

Pulsed electromagnetic field therapy, which has been more extensively studied in MS than static magnets, uses devices that produce pulsing, electromagnetic fields at a specific frequency. In one MS study, devices with a strong, pulsing magnetic field were placed on the spine. In other studies, small devices with weak, pulsing magnetic fields were placed on the legs on specific acupuncture points.

In four placebo-controlled clinical trials of pulsed electromagnetic therapy in MS three of these have involved weak magnetic fields, and one involved strong magnetic fields applied to the spine. In the study of strong magnetic fields applied to the spine, spasticity was found to be significantly decreased in the treated group compared to the placebo group. In the three studies with the weaker devices, beneficial effects on spasticity and improvement in pain, bladder function, hand function, fatigue, and quality of life were found in some studies. Given the variable findings and lack of rigor in some of these studies, further investigation is needed to clarify whether this therapy has any definite beneficial effects.

Short-term use of magnetic field therapy is usually well tolerated. The long-term effects of this treatment have not been investigated. Treatment with a strong magnet on the spine may produce dizziness and a band-like sensation around the torso. The weaker devices may cause headaches. Pregnant women and people with pacemakers or other electronic medical devices should consult with their physician before using these devices. Devices with a weak magnetic field are of low-moderate cost. Devices with a strong magnetic field are for experimental use and are not generally available.

Massage

Massage, one of the oldest forms of treatment, is a form of bodywork in which soft tissue is manipulated with pressure and traction. The common forms of massage in Western countries are derived from Swedish massage, which was developed by a Swedish physician in the nineteenth century.

In one study of massage therapy, twenty-four people with MS were assigned either to a control group that received "standard medical care" or to a massage treatment group that received standard medical care in combination with twice-weekly, in-home massage therapy. Relative to the start of the study, the treatment group exhibited less anxiety and depression after the first massage session and improvement in self-esteem, body image, "image of disease progression," and social functioning at the end of the five-week study. The results of this study are promising but not definitive. Larger studies with more well-matched groups and more rigorous study design are needed.

Massage is usually well tolerated. Minor side effects include headache, lethargy, and muscle pain. More serious side effects, such as bone fractures and bleeding into the liver, are possible but rare. Massage should be avoided or used with caution by people with the following conditions: clotted blood vessels (thrombosis), burns, skin infections, open wounds, bone fractures, osteoporosis, cancer, pregnancy, and heart disease. Massage is readily available and of low-moderate cost.

Reflexology

Reflexology is a type of bodywork in which manual pressure is applied to specific areas. These areas, which are usually on the feet but may also be on the hands and ears, are thought to correspond to specific organs and distant parts of the body. It is believed that pressure at specific reflexology sites improves energy flow to the corresponding body parts. This improved energy flow is claimed to improve health.

In one controlled study of reflexology, seventy-one people with MS were treated for eleven weeks with either reflexology or non-specific massage of the calf area. Relative to the control group, the people treated with reflexology exhibited significant improvement in paresthesias, urinary symptoms, and spasticity. Larger and more rigorous studies with lower dropout rates are needed.

Reflexology is generally well tolerated. Mild side effects include fatigue, foot pain, and changes in bowel and bladder function. Reflexology should be avoided or used with caution by people with bone or joint conditions of the feet and by those with other foot conditions such as gout, ulcers, and vascular disease.

Tai Chi

Tai chi is a traditional Chinese martial art that has been practiced for centuries in China. There has been recent interest in tai chi in some Western countries. Tai chi is characterized by a series of body postures that are linked by slow, graceful movements.

In one study, nineteen people with variable levels of MS disability were enrolled in an eight-week tai chi program. At the end of the program, there was improvement in walking speed and muscle stiffness, as well as in vitality, social and emotional functioning, and ability to carry out physical and emotional roles. Another study of sixteen people with MS used the tai chi principle of "mindfulness of movement," which involves developing moment-to-moment awareness of movement, breathing, and posture. Relative to the control group, which received "current available care," the treated group did not improve in balance but did improve in multiple MS-associated symptoms, as assessed by patients and by their relatives. Relative to pre-treatment, the treated group improved in balance. Larger and more rigorous studies are needed.

Tai chi is usually well tolerated. Mild side effects include strained muscles and joints. It may worsen MS-related fatigue. It should be avoided or used with caution by those with severe osteoporosis, acute low back pain, significant joint injuries, and bone fractures. Tai chi is low-moderate cost.

Yoga

Yoga is a mind-body approach that was developed in India thousands of years ago. It is derived from the Sanskrit word for *union* and is meant to unite the mind, body, and spirit. In *hatha yoga*, one of the more popular forms of yoga, the three main components are breathing, meditation, and posture.

In spite of yoga's popularity in some countries, there are very limited clinical studies of its effects in MS and other diseases. There is one well-designed, controlled trial of yoga in MS. In this six-month study, sixty-nine people with MS were randomized to a control group that received no intervention or to groups that were treated with conventional exercise or yoga. Relative to the control group, the yoga and conventional exercise groups had significant decreases in fatigue on the basis of two different measures. There were no consistent effects of yoga or conventional exercise on cognitive function or mood. It is not possible to determine whether yoga's effects on fatigue were due to the result of the yoga itself or resulted from other factors, such as a placebo response or benefits from being in a social setting.

Yoga is generally safe. In the clinical trial of yoga and MS, it was not associated with any serious adverse effects. Difficult postures or vigorous exercise should be avoided or done with caution by pregnant women, people with significant heart, lung, or bone conditions, or people with heat sensitivity, fatigue, and decreased balance. Yoga is a low-cost therapy, especially when it is done in groups.

Angioplasty of Neck Veins

In 2009 Dr. Paolo Zamboni presented a small, uncontrolled study of sixty-five patients that had what he called chronic cerebrospinal venous insufficiency (CCSVI), with narrowing or obstruction of neck veins he postulated would cause back pressure and reflux of blood into the nervous system. The treatment would then be to unblock the abnormal veins by a balloon inserted by catheter through the venous system. The balloon would be blown up to expand the vein, and then withdrawn. He had assessed the neck veins of normal people and a group of patients with other neurological conditions and said all MS patients had CCSVI, but none of the normal people or those with other neurological conditions. This caused great media attention and excitement in the MS community. There were immediate calls for this treatment to be made available.

Neurologists have been skeptical because there were no randomized clinical trials to substantiate the benefits and safety of the procedure and many studies soon after have failed to demonstrate the claims of Dr. Zamboni. There was also concern that Dr. Zamboni's claim was that early relapsing-remitting MS patients showed benefit, but those with secondary progressive or primary progressive MS did not benefit, the latter two groups were most of the patients who went for this therapy.

No study since has shown the dramatic results in the test or treatment that he showed. A Buffalo study shortly after Zamboni's initial presentation showed that only half of the MS patients had some evidence of obstruction in their neck veins, indicating half did not have this. More puzzling, almost half of the people with other neurological disease had some venous obstruction in their neck, and one out of four normal people had some obstruction to neck veins. This raised questions about whether it was a real disorder or not. Other studies showed that the positioning of the patient could alter the results and show obstruction, when another position did not. Also, later studies showed that evidence of some obstruction was less common at the beginning of the disease and more common later, suggesting it may be the result of having MS rather than a cause of the disease. Part of the Zamboni theory is that venous obstruction would cause increased pressure in the venous system within the brain and spinal cord, but a study with ophthalmodynamometry did not show any difference in the venous pressure in the central nervous system in thirty MS patients and thirty normal people.

Studies from England, Germany, Canada, Sweden, and the United States raised questions about the CCSVI concept as the studies did not show much difference between MS patients and normal people when neck veins were assessed by different procedures. Many clinical research groups feel the apparent neck obstruction is a reflection of how the studies are done, not a real obstruction, and that CCSVI is not a real condition. Also, the weight of evidence from many studies shows that patients often say they feel better but there is no objective evidence that their condition is measurably improved. In fact, a study from Texas suggested the MRIs had more lesions in the group who had the neck procedure performed compared to the sham-placebo group. There are many things to be learned about the CCSVI story. It seems clear that CCSVI is not the cause of MS, and many not even be a condition.

In the midst of all this confusion, conflicting results and unanswered questions, we are seeing claims by patients that some of their symptoms, especially fatigue, "brain fog," limb coldness, and numbness, may improve after having the procedure. Studies are being completed to answer further questions about diagnosis, treatment results, and follow-up results. It has been shown that many of the veins collapse after the procedure and the apparent benefit is lost. The current procedure often fails and the patients have a return of their symptoms after some months. To prevent the vein from collapsing, a stent could be put in, a procedure often used in arteries for coronary disease, but putting stents in veins has many risks and complications. In an artery the stent will stay fixed as arteries get smaller beyond the stent. In veins the stent can get loose as veins get bigger beyond the stent, and clotting around the stent is common as blood flow is slower and under less pressure than in arteries.

The major questions for patients and neurologists will only be answered by a large and well-designed randomized clinical trial that assesses a large range of subjective and objective measures of symptoms, MRI and neurological outcomes. Many such trials are now underway and others are in the design stage.

Carrying out clinical trials takes large numbers of patients and a large control group, and takes a long time if the trial is to demonstrate clinical symptoms and disability. Patients who were excited about the idea of CCSVI were frustrated by the length of time it would take to get the answers and wanted the therapy available before adequate randomized clinical trials, which are required before any drug would be approved for therapy. Unfortunately, this has resulted in a tension between patients and the clinicians, MS organizations, and even governments who were portrayed as delaying their ability to get the procedure.

It is expensive and the amount depends on the country where it is being done, travel, and follow-up. There are known risks and complications, including collapse of the veins, clotting, stroke, and death. The detailed degree of risk is uncertain as many of the centers do not conduct follow-up studies.

CHAPTER 6

Practical Guidelines for Living with Multiple Sclerosis

There are many things you can do to stay as healthy as possible, take control of your life, and cope with the challenges that MS may bring. The disease should not be in control—*you* are in control of your life, your attitudes, your relationships, your approach to problems, your interests, and your activities.

This chapter discusses some things you should do and some things you should not do. For example, you should get more information about MS; you should make sure you have an opportunity to ask questions about the disease; you should exercise; you should try to live a normal, active life, adapting to any limitations; you should work to improve your relationships; you should express a positive attitude; and you should have regular medical assessments.

There are things you should not do. Do not withdraw from life and friends; do not stop exercising; do not expose yourself to a hot environment; do not try every treatment that you hear about without first getting reliable information about the scientific evidence, possible benefits, and side effects; and do not feel ashamed or diminished because you have MS.

Where Can I Learn More About MS?

Many things are known about MS, and many advances are being made. There are many unanswered questions, but it is important to learn more about the questions that are being asked by researchers and the theories that are being tested.

One of the best initial sources of information is the Multiple Sclerosis Society, which can be accessed through their website in each country. They can be contacted directly as well. In the United States, call 800-344-4867 to reach the National MS Society; in Canada call 800-268-7582. Other sources of information are the Multiple Sclerosis Association of America (MSAA; www.msassociation.org) at 800-532-7667, and the Multiple Sclerosis Foundation (www.msf .org) at 800-225-6495.

What Should Others Know About MS?

It is important for your family, friends, and coworkers to understand MS. Initially you may feel that you do not want others to know that you have MS. That is understandable, but it is essential to tell the people you love, and others when necessary, so that they can understand and help you deal with the disease. Most people with MS are pleased and surprised at how supportive and understanding others are when they are informed. Many people may have guessed that something was wrong but did not know what to do or say. Until they know the truth, employers may not understand your need to take time off or to rest, and they may think you are not working well. Decisions to inform should be made on an individual basis, but, in general, disclosure is a good idea.

Once family and friends are aware of your diagnosis, they might benefit from literature that would allow them to better understand MS.

In particular, your family should understand your symptoms and problems so they can be helpful and supportive. This is not possible if they are unaware of your MS and how it makes you feel.

Who Can Answer My Questions?

It is important to have your concerns addressed and your questions answered. Often people are afraid that they might ask too many questions or that their questions might not be clear. Make a list of the questions you want to ask. Bring the questions to your physician or nurse on your next visit or call the MS Society. You probably will find that they are questions most people ask and that they are not new to the staff. If there is no clear answer to a question, it is important to find that out as well. Each new piece of information will add to your overall understanding of MS.

What Can I Learn from Other People Who Have MS?

People with MS soon learn that it is a common neurological disorder and that there are many others in their community who have the same disease. It often helps to talk to others who share the challenges and problems of coping with MS, but there are some cautions.

> *You cannot compare yourself with others in terms of the type of disease, the course, or the symptoms. Multiple sclerosis is an individual disease, and you probably will find that the features of your MS are quite different from those of the next person.*

It may seem puzzling that there are so many individual patterns for the disease, but that is actually fairly common in other diseases as well. The variety of symptoms of MS is great, so the variations in individuals are great as well.

One way that people with MS can benefit from each other is in self-help or support groups. These take various forms, but they usually are small groups that meet in homes or in community facilities to talk about and better understand MS. The object is always to take a positive approach and to take control over everything that you can manage so that you can help yourself and others. The MS Society has information on support groups and MS centers often sponsor them. It is important to select a group lead by someone who truly knows MS and can make your experience with the group a positive learning one. A group without direction and without a positive focus can be a negative experience.

When Is Information Not Helpful?

Misinformation is not helpful and can cause much trouble and distress, not to mention wasted time and money. If someone says that mercury in dental fillings causes MS, check it out from those who know—staff at the MS Society, someone in the MS clinic in your area, or your physician—but do not go to the dentist and have your fillings removed. If someone tells you that ginseng cures MS, check it out. If someone says there is a doctor in a clinic somewhere who has a cure for MS, call the MS Society, not your travel agent. Although there is good information on the Internet, there are some sites and chat rooms that provide misinformation. It is sometimes hard to see which are reliable and which are not. So choose your Internet sources wisely and always question what you read.

What About My Activities?

People with MS should lead normal and active lives within the limitations of their symptoms. This means that we encourage activity more than rest and staying active and involved rather than withdrawing and dropping out. We want people to remain productive and working. It is understandable that symptoms and problems may make this harder for you, taking more time and energy, but it is still better to do it than not to do it.

People with MS are happiest and at their best when they live as normally as possible and carry out the activities they enjoy. There are no absolute limitations—if you feel like walking in a march, running a race, or climbing a mountain, and do not have symptoms and problems that limit you, go for it! Unfortunately, MS does cause symptoms that may limit activities to some extent. It requires adjustment so that you can continue to do as much as you can, in the time you need, and in the way you can manage. If you work at managing your problems, coping with any limitations, and keeping a positive attitude, not only can you do many of the things in life you want to do, but also you may accomplish much more than others without MS, as they often do not use these positive skills to deal with life.

What About Exercise?

Simply put, exercise is good for everyone. When the diagnosis of MS is made, you should set about getting yourself in the best shape that you can, both mentally and physically, in order to manage any challenges that come with the disease. We all benefit from regular exercise, and it is even more important for the person with MS. If fatigue is a problem, you should arrange your exercise for times when fatigue is less bothersome, schedule it in periods with breaks, or redesign the type and pattern of exercise so that you can still do it.

In general, the best exercise is one that you enjoy so that you will continue to always do it, not just because it is good for you. Exercise should be a lifetime habit for all of us, including people with MS, even if the exercise program needs to be modified at times. Try to involve others in exercise as well. Exercise programs in the community have a tendency to motivate you to participate regularly; they also have an enjoyable social aspect.

Can I Overdo It?

Many MS patients worry that overdoing things might cause attacks of MS and worsen the disease. Friends and family often tell MS patients to rest most of the time. This is not good advice.

There is no evidence that exercising or even overdoing work and activities have any deleterious effect on MS. True, it may make you feel tired for the next day or so, but there is no evidence that it worsens your MS. Some people "push through" their fatigue, which also may make them tired the next day but does no long-term harm.

It might be tempting to blame over-activity for the development of a new attack of MS or a new symptom, especially if it happened a day or a few days later, but a careful accounting of strenuous events, stressful events, and the occurrence of attacks would show that this is probably coincidental. Do not worry about activity; be reasonable, keep active, and do what you can.

How Much Should I Rest?

Because fatigue is a major problem for many people with MS, a reasonable balance between maintaining your normal activities and taking brief rests is appropriate. People usually find their own balance of activity and rest, and in this way they keep up their activity, work, and other responsibilities.

It is important to recognize that the fatigue in MS is not "normal" tiredness that follows too little sleep or a long, hard day though people with MS are not exempt from that kind of tiredness as well. When you are experiencing fatigue, it is important to take the time to examine all that you are doing in a day to see if what you expect of yourself is reasonable. The fatigue in MS is usually felt as different from the normal fatigue everyone experiences; it is unrelated to the amount of sleep and activity. It can occur in waves and may seem overwhelming at times. If you are experiencing MS fatigue, examine the hour of the day and change your schedule so that you are not doing the most important things when you know that fatigue is greatest. Adapting the level of activities is often successful, and some medications also may be helpful (see Chapter 4).

Do not rest too much. *Activity* is a more important watchword than rest in MS.

What About Stress?

Everyone experiences stress in their lives, and being given a diagnosis of MS is certainly stressful. Having to see yourself and your life in a different light, with greater uncertainty, is stressful. But marriage, raising children, doing our jobs, and the "daily-ness" of life also bring stress. The central point is not whether stress is present in your life (it almost always is), but your response to it. People can, and do, react differently. Some see stress as a problem to be solved. Some respond emotionally, collapsing in tears, becoming depressed, or lashing out angrily at others. Some are initially upset, but then set about overcoming or dealing with the stress. Others do not believe it is possible to deal with it and give up. It is not the stress; it is our reaction to it that makes the difference.

When people react to stress in a nonproductive way, they often state that anyone would react the same way. That isn't true because in the same situation, different people respond differently. Fortunately, by analyzing such events, you can learn how to react more positively. It is not easy and sometimes requires counseling, but a person who reacts ineffectively to stress can learn how to respond better. It does mean that you must recognize that your responses could be more productive before you can work at it or seek help.

Can I Develop Better Coping Skills?

We all have certain patterns of coping. Some of us react more intellectually to problems and stresses, while others react more emotionally. Most of us have a combination of the two; it is the balance of intellectual problem-solving responses and emotional responses that is important.

It is natural to feel upset when something stressful happens. However, it is not normal for that to be the only response. There is a point at which we must think clearly and objectively about what the stress is all about, how we can analyze it, and how we can most effectively deal with it. That combines the appropriate emotional and problem-solving aspect. You can improve these coping skills by improving their components. When a stressful event has passed, you can analyze how well you responded—whether your emotional response was appropriate and balanced, and whether the steps you took were the most effective ones to deal with the problem. Such analysis often gives you a different perspective, particularly if it is done in an honest fashion and enables you to see how you could respond more effectively the next time.

How Can I Maintain a Positive Attitude?

The most important factor in dealing with MS—or any challenge in life—is a mature, positive, and good-humored attitude whenever possible.

Some people struggle harder than others. There is no question that a positive attitude is of great importance because a negative person cannot tolerate very much adversity. MS does not make you positive or negative; you already had an approach to life before you developed the disease. MS can challenge your approach, your positivity, and your good humor, however, so it is important to make an even greater effort to overcome difficulties in a way that makes you feel good and improves your relationships. People like to be around those who are positive and good humored. We can understand those who are negative and turn their frustration on others, but they do not manage well, are more unhappy, and do not learn to take control of the things they can manage.

It is important to practice being positive and good natured and cheerful. That may sound false, but when you smile and talk in a positive manner, you feel better and others feel better. Attitude is so important and you can practice seeing things and speaking in a positive manner. It will change how you see your world and your situation.

What About My Relationships?

Good relationships are important to us all, and they become even more important when we have difficult challenges to overcome. In taking control of your health and your future you should strengthen your relationships. It may seem simplistic, but it actually is one of the most important things you can do. It has a positive effect on you when you do everything you can to improve your relationships with your spouse, your children, your family, your friends, and everyone with whom you come in contact. Our relationships with others are central to our happiness and state of well-being, and it is rewarding to continue to improve them. There is a large body of research evidence showing that better outcomes in MS are related to a strong support system of family, friends, and caregivers.

Should I Tell People I Have MS?

It is natural that you may have felt uncertain about telling people— even your family or close friends—when you first were told that you have MS. It is hard to recognize that something about yourself has changed, and it is worrisome to think that it might affect your relationships and how people regard you. Eventually you will come to recognize that you are still the same person, that the people who love you will continue to love you and support you, and that others generally are understanding and helpful. Sometimes they may try to be too helpful, as most people don't want relationships to change. All of these feelings plus some embarrassment about "having an illness" make many people want to hide the diagnosis. They think, "maybe if I pretend the problem doesn't exist, it won't exist."

It is a good rule to be honest and open in our relationships and interactions. Of course, like all health matters, the fact that you have MS is a private and confidential matter, so who you confide in is a personal choice. It is common to keep the information within a small circle initially, especially because everything may be calm and stable for many years. A problem begins to develop when symptoms cause difficulties that are visible to others, but they have not been made aware that you have a health problem. At that point, others may wonder, worry, and speculate about what is happening, and their speculation can be more harmful than the truth.

It also is worth considering that people feel excluded and not trusted when they are kept in the dark yet know that something is being kept secret. There are some instances when keeping a medical problem a secret can be a serious offense or can cause serious problems.

For example, you cannot lie about having a medical problem when answering questions on insurance forms or other official documents. There are only a few instances when it is proper to ask such questions, but in such instances, you must answer truthfully.

What Happens When It Is Hot?

Most, but not all, people with MS find that they are heat sensitive. They notice that they become weak or dizzy, or even feel sick, in a hot bath, on a hot humid day, or in a warm environment. They also notice the opposite—they feel better and function better when it is cooler, when they are swimming in cool water, or when they move from a warm room to a cool room.

Remyelinated and partially damaged nerve fibers may function less well when body temperature is elevated and, conversely, the nerves function better when temperature is lowered. This tends to be a transient phenomenon that does not produce a lasting effect. However, it can produce marked weakness, and people often describe themselves as feeling like a "dishrag" or "wiped out" on a hot day. This response to heat was once the basis of the *hot bath test*, which was used as a test for MS before modern diagnostic tests were available. Although it is suggestive of MS, it is not accurate enough to be an important test.

You may wonder whether becoming weak in a hot environment will make the disease worse, but the phenomenon is transient and disappears as soon as you cool off. We do recommend that you avoid a warm environment whenever possible because you will feel less well, function less well, and have more symptoms when it is very warm. Air conditioning often is required in summer months to maintain reasonable temperature control and is considered medically necessary for tax purposes (a letter from your physician is needed). Cool drinks are also helpful—get in the habit of carrying one with you. The fluids will help your bladder and bowel function as well. Cooling scarves and other cooling equipment may be helpful as well (see Chapter 4). Avoid sunbathing, saunas, and hot tubs.

Should I Change My Diet?

The dietary approach to the management of MS has a long history. It is difficult to perform clinical trials on diets, but there was interest and some suggestion of a positive response from studies of diets that are low in animal fats (essentially a low-cholesterol diet) and with a supplement of a vegetable oil such as sunflower seed oil or evening primrose oil. A few of these studies showed some positive benefit but one large study showed no benefit. There also was some suggestion that people with early and mild disease benefit the most. Many people use the simple approach to diet of lowering the amount of animal fat and supplementing it with a vegetable oil because it is a healthy diet and everyone in the family can potentially benefit from it. Many more complex diets have been recommended in MS, which have little logic or justification and are so complicated that people give them up after a short time (see the discussion on diet in Chapter 5).

The most important points are to stick to a balanced, healthy diet, maintain normal weight, and limit your intake of animal fat. This is a good dietary recommendation for everyone.

Should I Sleep More?

How much sleep you need is based on your own normal pattern. Some people require eight or nine hours a night, whereas others require only five or six hours. The average is seven and one-half hours of sleep, and the measure of effectiveness is how rested you feel in the morning. You should not change your sleep pattern because you have MS. Since fatigue is a major problem for many people, there is a tendency to think that you will be less fatigued if you sleep more.

However, even with normal or greater sleep hours, you will still tend to feel tired during the day if fatigue is due to MS. Surprisingly, over-sleeping often makes people feel more tired. It is worth remembering that many factors can decrease the quality of sleep, including alcohol and many drugs.

What If I Need Surgery?

The answer to this question is simple. If you need surgery and there are good indications for surgery, you should have it. If you do not need surgery, you should not have it. This is a good rule whether you have MS or not. There does not appear to be any increased risk to people with MS who undergo surgery. In the past, there was concern that the stress of surgery might precipitate MS attacks, but the number of attacks of MS that occur in those circumstances is the same as that which would be expected in an average population of people with the disease, and no more. This is in keeping with the previous point that there is little evidence that stressful events precipitate attacks of MS, whether they involve surgery, anesthesia, trauma, or major life events. The most important rule is to be assured that surgery is truly indicated and necessary.

Is Pregnancy a Risk?

The relationship between MS and pregnancy has been carefully studied. Pregnancy does not increase the incidence of attacks of MS and in the final trimester, the number of attacks is reduced. Studies indicate that the likelihood of an attack of MS decreases by up to 70 percent during this period. However, there are more attacks in the six months following delivery than would be expected in a six-month period (see discussion of hormones during pregnancy in Chapter 10). Those episodes should be treated and managed like any other episode of MS. Pregnancy has no long-term effects on disability or disease progression.

Two other aspects of pregnancy and child rearing must be considered. First, there is a small, but real, genetic risk for MS in a family— about 5 percent for a first-degree relative. This is greater than the risk in the normal population, but it clearly is low. More significantly, raising a child is a life-long responsibility, and people with MS must recognize that their health during the time that they will need to carry out this responsibility may be uncertain. For example, one cannot predict health status in ten or fifteen years. This probably is the major factor that governs the decision about having a child. Recognizing the risks and problems, each couple must determine for themselves as this very personal decision.

Will MS Affect My Sex Life?

Because MS affects the central nervous system and the nerves that control various functions in the body, the complex and sensitive control system for sexual function also can be affected. Early in the disease there may be no physical effect on sexual function, but the enjoyment of sex may be affected by your emotional state. Worries, depression, or altered feelings about yourself can affect your relationship with others and the normal emotions associated with sexuality. Thus, sexual function may be affected by psychologic factors, and this possibility needs to be considered. More often there is a physiologic basis for the difficulties, seen in conjunction with bladder and bowel symptoms. For men, the most common problem is achieving or maintaining an erection, which can be helped by medication such as sildenafil citrate (Viagra), tadalafil (Cialis), avanafil (Stendra), or vardenafil (Levitra, Staxyn). Women may experience decreased vaginal lubrication, which can be accommodated by synthetic lubricating products, such as Astroglide or K-Y Jelly. Never use petroleum jelly (Vaseline). If you experience sexual problems, talk with your physician or health care professional and do not suffer in silence. There are informative pamphlets from the MS societies on sexuality in MS.

What About Driving?

Driving is only a problem when symptoms or limitations make it risky or unacceptably difficult. Vertigo, double vision, or a temporary loss of vision would not permit you to drive safely. Problems with leg weakness, spasticity, or incoordination limit rapid and accurate use of brake and accelerator pedals and make driving unsafe. It may be possible to return to driving when symptoms improve, but it is wise to depend on the assessment of your physician when there is any question about this. Most rehabilitation facilities can assess whether a person can drive safely.

When a problem is more long standing and renders driving unsafe, it may be possible to adapt the controls on the vehicle to allow a person to drive. The most common adaptation is to covert foot pedals to hand controls.

Although a person may be anxious to continue driving and willing to take some chances, feeling that they are "all right to drive," greater consideration must be given to others who may be at risk, including passengers, pedestrians, and other drivers.

Should I Move?

Some people with MS ask if it would be helpful if they moved to another area because they have read that the incidence of MS varies in different parts of the world, that it is more common in temperate climates, and that it is rare in very hot climates, such as near the Equator. The answer is no. In fact, they might find the heat a problem because it tends to make people with MS feel worse. We also believe that the geographic patterns of MS incidence probably have other explanations, and have had the effect earlier in life. There is no evidence that moving to another area once you have the disease will help.

Will I Be Different?

It is natural to wonder how MS will change you. Young people see themselves as healthy and perfect and do not visualize themselves with a serious and chronic disease. When you are given a diagnosis of a medical condition, it is natural to begin to think of yourself differently, and you may have to readjust your self-concept. You are still *you*, but it requires you to see that a different element has entered your life. Many things change as you go through life—some good, some not so good. What is necessary is a positive approach to challenges and determination to move ahead. This may be easier said than done so don't feel guilty if your doctor suggests some counseling to get you started and give you support.

What About Other Questions I May Have?

This chapter could not possibly cover all the questions you may have, but covers some of the most common questions I hear from patients. You will have many more, and they should be asked of your physician, other health care professionals, or staff at the MS Society. It is always better to ask a question even if you are uncertain about exactly how to ask it or if you think it sounds "silly" than to wonder or worry in silence.

We recommend the book *Multiple Sclerosis: The Questions You Have, The Answers You Need* as a more detailed guide to many of your questions (see Additional Reading).

CHAPTER 7

Coping with Multiple Sclerosis

Being diagnosed with MS can create turmoil in every area of a person's life. In some ways, life will never be quite the same again. Even in the absence of impairment, the worry—or effort to camouflage worry—is always there. The diagnosis often precipitates a roller coaster ride of emotions. The time following diagnosis can be challenging and confusing. This chapter helps you to bring perspective to the emotional turmoil and helps you think about ways to ease the distress and continue with your life.

The Crisis of Diagnosis

People have a variety of reactions when they are given a diagnosis of MS. Some experience a combination of fear and confusion when first confronted with the news. These feelings may be quickly replaced by denial, a refusal to believe that this could possibly be happening. "There must be some mistake!" is a common reaction to the diagnosis, often followed quickly by feelings of anger and resentment. Lisa's story provides an example of some of these feelings. When asked about her initial experience with the diagnosis of MS, Lisa (then 19 years old), replied:

> *I was having a multitude of symptoms that I didn't understand, such as numbness in my feet. I was having trouble feeling the ground when I was walking. I couldn't see very well out of my left eye—it was almost like looking through an oily film. A whole bunch of odd things were happening that I didn't understand. When I finally got the diagnosis, I was really scared. I didn't know what MS was or what would happen to me. I was afraid of the whole thing.*

> *Later I was angry—very angry. Then I decided there was no way I could really have this disease. In fact, my parents and I were second-guessing the doctors—going from one to another asking what was wrong with me. All I could think of was that can in the grocery store that you throw your loose change into—you know, the one with the picture of someone in a wheelchair. It was probably a good year before I even started to accept the fact that I have MS. There was no way I could have it—I'm too active and I do so many things. And I can't stop doing them.*

The diagnosis actually brings a sense of relief for some people, especially those who had disturbing but vague symptoms for a long time, sometimes years, but were given many explanations that didn't seem to provide an adequate explanation. After being told it was due to stress, a pinched nerve, or some vague condition, it is a relief to finally know the answer. They knew there was something wrong, and the lack of an explanation, or feeling doctors must think "it is all in my mind," was more stressful than having a diagnosis. There may also be a sense of relief if the person was worried about something worse, such as a brain tumor. Another sense of relief can come from now knowing how to deal with a definite answer.

Jim, who was diagnosed with MS in 2004 after a frustrating search for some answers, spoke about fear and relief at finally learning his diagnosis:

It took me a year to get a diagnosis. I was scared to death when I heard "MS." I didn't even know what MS was. But I was also relieved. When you're used to not having a label for all the strange things that are going on and suddenly the problem is identified for you, that alone is a relief— all this finally has a name.

Regardless of the initial emotional response, the diagnosis of MS creates a crisis for the individual and the entire family. The person who has been diagnosed may experience a sense of isolation despite efforts of family members to offer support. Lisa mentioned this experience:

Even though people wanted to help, I was the one who had to learn to live with it and had to learn what I needed to do to live with it. You have to make your choice of how you're going to live your life. You have to do it because it's your disease and nobody can do it for you or make it go away.

Family members are also immersed in their own concerns about their loved one, but also about the future and the impact that MS will have on their lives. The positive aspect of this type of crisis (if you can even imagine one) is that it provides an opportunity to assess future plans and a powerful motivation to take actions that support those plans. There is an opportunity to affirm the values and strengths of the individual and the family and all the good things that remain intact in spite of MS. In order to go forward, it is important to know that you can successfully move through the difficult emotions and continue to pursue your goals and dreams. A professional counselor—such as a psychologist or social worker—can be a helpful ally to the person with MS and family members in working toward a positive outlook for the future.

The Adjustment Process

The initial reactions to the diagnosis of MS often give way to a feeling of sadness related to the addition of a serious chronic illness to one's identity and self-image. Chronic illness forces each person to confront the frailty and vulnerability of the human condition in a personal way. There is also the concern that there may be a negative attitude by society to people with a chronic disease. This process involves grieving for your former self-image and integrating the realities of MS into one's identity. Sadness, anger at the disease, and self-absorption also might be experienced during this time.

Grieving is necessary for a person to move forward, just as it is following the loss of a loved one. Unlike the grieving we associate with the loss of someone, the grieving process in chronic illness tends to ebb and flow of symptoms and physical changes over time. Grief may be postponed, but usually not completely avoided. Sometimes these feelings may be channeled inappropriately, such as anger at one's spouse or children or at health professionals who cannot cure the illness. It is important for everyone involved to understand this grieving process and to show understanding and support.

The period of intense grieving may last from a few weeks to several months, with gradually diminishing intensity. As it subsides, at least for the time being, one can again begin to focus on and enjoy special relationships and daily activities. Ideally, there is a gradual acknowledgment of the permanence of MS in one's life, while maintaining a sense of continuity between the past and the future as well as a commitment to maximizing the quality of life.

Depressive feelings may occur as part of the initial grieving process or in response to subsequent changes or losses imposed by the illness. Over the course of the disease, however, individuals with MS are at greater than average risk for depression. Often the person can get through this, particularly when they clarify their understanding, become more positive about how they are going to move ahead and deal with any issues. It is important, however, to recognize when this is not working and the person stays in a state of depression that is affecting his or her life and normal functioning, and therapy with counseling or medication may be necessary. Symptoms of significant depression include ongoing and pervasive sadness, loss of interest in or enjoyment of important activities and relationships, feelings of hopelessness and despair, sometimes including suicidal feelings or thoughts, and changes in sleeping and eating patterns. Family members may notice some of these changes and point them out to the doctor when they accompany the person at their next visit to the doctor. Intervention is recommended if any of these symptoms continue for an extended period of time or seem to be worsening. It is important to realize that relief from depression is readily available. Seeking help for this problem demonstrates an understanding of its significance, not personal weakness or deficiency.

Jim comments on his experience with depression:

I was pretty depressed, so I went to see a psychologist. She was connected with a rehabilitation facility, so her primary interest was working with people who are chronically ill or disabled to help them find comfortable ways of living and thinking about themselves. It was a perfect match because that's just what I needed at that point.

One hallmark of MS that is most troubling and challenging for patients is the unpredictability of the disease course and the uncertainties related to future ability/disability. That sense of control you had over your life is shaken. Questions that almost everyone faces include: What symptoms and impairments might occur? When will new symptoms appear? When will they go away Or will they go away? Amy, who was diagnosed eight years ago, addressed this issue:

I think not knowing what will happen is the hardest thing for people when they're diagnosed with MS. They totally freak out and wonder, "what's this disease going to do to me?" They have to realize that what happens to someone else is not necessarily going to happen to them. And if it does, well, you will have to deal with it.

Flexibility is a key element in living with the unpredictability of MS. Goals need to be assessed and revised, with a "plan for the worst, hope for the best" outlook. A college student named Leslie was pursuing a career in horticulture, which necessitated spending a fair amount of time in greenhouses. Her early symptoms included heat sensitivity, with temporary blurred vision and extreme fatigue when she was exposed to warm temperatures. Although this problem remitted, any future recurrence would have prevented Leslie from performing her job. After careful thought, she switched to teaching, an occupation that heat sensitivity and other possible MS symptoms would not prevent her from continuing. Similarly, the purchase of a new home should involve consideration of issues of mobility and accessibility. Many people with MS are not significantly bothered by problems with walking. However, since mobility impairment is a problem at some point for many people with MS, it is simply good planning to consider this possibility when choosing a home, even while being reasonably optimistic that serious walking difficulties will not occur.

Resilience

The ability to overcome adversity and loss and come back even stronger, having learned from the experience is called resilience. Everyone experiences adversity in life, the loss of a loved one, failure in business, loss of a job, or breakdown of a marriage. The hope is that the person can at some stage step back, examine the situation, and reconfigure life, having learned some lessons.

Anyone is capable of this, but particularly those who have a positive personality, have a positive sense of themselves, a tendency to evaluate circumstances realistically, manage strong emotions, are effective at solving problems, and communicate well with others.

Some of the most prominent successful individuals are winners because they failed so many times (Steve Jobs, Winston Churchill, Oprah Winfrey, Thomas Edison, Michael Jordan, and Martin Luther King, Jr.). They were upset by the losses and failures, but could reassess their situation and come back stronger.

Managing the stresses and losses also requires you to be in the best general health, so have regular exercise and sleep, and mental relaxation. It requires you to be honest in your evaluation of yourself, your circumstances, and the options. It is helpful to have good communication with family and friends.

At the time of a stressful event it is tempting to feel there is no way to deal with it. Examine your responses and how you could have done things better. Don't make excuses or justify behaviors, but think about improving a better outcome for you and for others. Practice being positive. Examine and work at the positive things in your life. Don't dwell on things you can't do, but what you can do. Practice being more understanding and forgiving as resentments and anger sap your energy and make it hard to be happy and positive as you strive for a positive recovery from a difficult time.

Coping Strategies

Coping strategies reflect an individual's personality and attitudes and the way the individual interacts with people and events. By adulthood, personal strategies have been selected and refined through an unconscious process; most of us do not consciously choose and evaluate our coping mechanisms. How we respond to issues in life is, to a great extent, developed early in childhood, but we can modify our responses if they are not helpful or constructive. We can assess how we deal with people, stresses, and life issues honestly and critically and accentuate the good patterns and train ourselves to modify and reduce personal reactions that are unhelpful and negative. The following are examples of two types of strategies.

Denial

Denial is ignoring or minimizing the seriousness of the situation. Intermittent denial may be useful in the early stages of adapting to MS because it enables people to deal with the immediate symptoms they are experiencing without having to contemplate all the possible problems that may occur in the future. Denial is *not* useful if these potential problems are ignored when making important life-planning decisions such as buying a home or making career decisions. One of the most serious consequences of continued denial is avoidance of treatments, as intellectually people know they have MS but emotionally deny there is really anything wrong.

Denial can also interfere with obtaining optimal health care. A denial of a well-established diagnosis of MS can lead to a search for any other possible explanation resulting in unnecessary tests, unnecessary surgery, and delays in therapy that should be started early in the disease.

Intellectualization

Intellectualization is focusing on available factual information to the exclusion of feelings and other psychological issues. A certain amount of intellectualization makes it possible for people to learn about the disease, assess its impact on their daily lives, and make use of their problem-solving abilities to meet the challenges imposed by MS. Intellectualization becomes excessive when it consumes enormous amounts of energy; some people expend so much effort collecting and analyzing information that they have little or no energy left to deal with their emotional reactions to the disease or with the feelings and reactions of those around them.

Looking at these two examples, the strengths and weaknesses inherent in some coping strategies can be seen. Denial is useful in allowing a person to get on with his or her life, but it is detrimental if it interferes with obtaining optimal treatment or with life-planning issues. Intellectualization is useful in obtaining essential information, but it is harmful when it is used as a means to block feelings about the disease that should be expressed. At the same time refusing to learn anything about the disease can be equally problematic. One needs to be able to address symptoms that may be due to MS and report them to their doctor to be addressed. The blocking of emotional awareness and expression can interfere with long-range coping efforts.

Interpersonal difficulties may arise when two people who live together and must cope with MS have conflicting coping styles. A person who copes by talking through feelings and events or by reading all the literature on MS may encounter resistance and even anger from a partner who is trying desperately to maintain denial as a way of dealing with the disease. In some situations, counseling is useful to help a couple or family members recognize each other's coping styles and provide mutual support.

Educate Yourself About MS

People with MS have indicated in National Multiple Sclerosis Society surveys that information about the disease and its effects is their most important need. Education about MS is available through a number of sources, primarily MS health care providers and the U.S., Canadian, and other national MS societies (see the Resources chapter). Keep in mind, however, that adults can choose to learn in a variety of ways and may choose to do so in different settings or at different times. For some, devouring every available piece of written material is the most desirable strategy. These individuals compare different sources of information, analyzing and sorting varied opinions, to create a personal perspective. The result is a sense of "ownership" of the information and its gradual integration into personal philosophy and decisions about day-to-day activities. Other people prefer a group setting that provides opportunities for the immediate testing of new ideas and feedback from peers and/or professionals.

Such group educational programs are widely available through the U.S., Canadian, and other national MS societies. The National Multiple Sclerosis Society in the United States has a mail program called "Knowledge Is Power" for people who have been recently diagnosed with MS. The program consists of a series of modules on topics of interest sent on a predetermined schedule to people who request this service. This mail series can be obtained by calling 1-800-FIGHT-MS. These publications are also available in Canada (416-922-6065). The Multiple Sclerosis Association of America and the Multiple Sclerosis Foundation also have excellent booklets of information that they make available for the asking. Each of these organizations has websites with good, unbiased information to access on the Internet as well. You'll find their web addresses in the Resources chapter.

Another component of the educational process relates to reports of possible treatments or "the cure" for MS. Given the variability and unpredictability of the illness over time, it is not surprising that diverse therapies have been heralded as having a significant impact on MS. When symptoms remit—as they frequently do quite naturally over the course of the disease—whatever treatment or activity is being used at the time is given credit for the improvement. Since dramatic improvement and long periods of remission are common occurrences in MS, even without any therapy, it is important to be prudently skeptical when evaluating therapies that claim to be of benefit. Only those treatments that have been evaluated for safety and efficacy in carefully designed and controlled scientific studies provide documentation of benefit. Other therapies are "experimental," meaning the benefits and risks have not yet been fully determined. There are also many suggested therapies, generally outside the usual medical interventions and called "complementary" or "alternative" therapies, that should also be carefully evaluated (see Chapters 6 and 11). Some of these claim a boost to the immune system and are not appropriate for people with MS, who already have an overly active immune system. Any non–physician-prescribed therapy that claims to reduce MS disease activity or any therapy that claims to cure MS should be avoided. Chapter 6 addresses unconventional therapies as does *Complementary and Alternative Medicine and Multiple Sclerosis* by Allen Bowling (see Additional Reading). Chapter 11 addresses the importance of clinical trials to clarify the safety and benefits of any potential therapy for MS.

Choosing Your Health Care Providers

The choice of health care providers is a critical decision relative to long-term management issues. People with MS generally have a normal or nearly normal life expectancy, and management of the disease is a lifelong process. The physician who manages the symptoms and disease course will interact with the other physicians involved in your health care, such as your internist, gynecologist/obstetrician, cardiologist, or any other medical specialist whose services you might require during your lifetime. Members of your chosen health care team will also provide you on an ongoing basis with information that you will need to make important life decisions relating, for example, to job choices, family planning, or the selection of an MS treatment option. Choose your health care providers carefully. Investigate your physician's board certification (neurology, family practice, or internal medicine), experience with MS, hospital or medical center affiliation, and reputation in the community. In most cases, you will need to have a relationship with an internist or family physician to monitor your general health and serve as your "primary care provider," and a neurologist to manage your MS. It is important to remember that though it is easy to blame MS for anything that happens to you after your diagnosis, MS does not exempt you from any other health problems. The local chapter (United States) or division (Canada) of the Multiple Sclerosis Society, can suggest physicians in the community who have experience in the management of MS or, if none is available locally, they will identify MS specialists within the broader geographic region.

Support Networks

Family and friends provide the major support for the person with MS. Their caring and concern are vital, especially during the difficult times following diagnosis or when a flare-up of symptoms occurs. A "sorting out" of friends and relatives may be necessary because not all people with a close relationship are able to be supportive in the same way. One person may be comfortable listening to concerns and providing emotional support, while another may find it easier to assist with more concrete activities, such as a ride to the doctor's office. Unfortunately, some friends may not be able to deal with chronic disease. Another friend or relative may be a great problem solver, helpful in finding solutions or identifying resources in troublesome situations.

At the same time, a person's ability to help should not be too narrowly or rigidly determined, especially without discussing it with him or her. It is important for all those who provide support to know how important their contributions are to the person with MS.

People with MS may find it especially helpful to talk with others who have the disease. This interaction will help to demonstrate that people with MS do indeed continue productive and satisfying lives despite the intrusion of the disease.

Many chapters of the National MS Society have "peer support" programs that train selected individuals with MS to be helpful to people who have questions about the disease. They are available to answer questions, discuss issues, and relate their personal MS successes and failures. In some areas, the peer is available for a telephone conversation; in other areas, the person may also be available at the local MS center on certain days. Amy commented on her experience with a peer support person:

> *Having that one-on-one interaction, having someone to talk to who understands, who has gone through similar experiences—that was really important to me. She was a source of strength and kept helping my self-image to stay in shape.*

Some people find a group setting most helpful because they can benefit from the experiences of a number of people with MS. Group members also feel good about the group interaction and support, which is much like a family support network. In an MS support group, MS temporarily feels "normal" because it is the common experience of all members. This normalization of MS is extremely supportive of the overall adjustment process. Instead of feeling isolated, the person in a support group sees MS as one component of a full and diverse life, which can be managed with an understanding of the disease, support of family, friends, health professionals, and peers with MS. Some support groups are led by a counseling professional such as a psychologist, or social worker, or MS nurse while others are "self-help" and are led by one of the group members.

To find a support group near you, or perhaps a telephone group, call 1-800-FIGHT-MS in the United States and 1-800-268-7582 in Canada. If you receive your care in an MS center, there may be support groups associated with your center.

Wellness Orientation

In contrast to a *disease orientation*, which focuses on minimizing the impact of the chronic disease on all aspects of your life, a *wellness approach* looks at achieving the positive state of maximal health despite the presence of a chronic illness. Wellness is a balanced state of positive well-being in mind, body, emotions, and spirit. This model encompasses interpersonal relationships as well as relationships with the environment, the community, and society in general. The wellness orientation is comprehensive in its promotion of mind-body unity within the individual, as well as integration of the individual within the community and society as a whole.

A practical example of a wellness orientation is the practice of aerobic and general conditioning exercises, which have an orientation different from that of traditional physical therapy designed primarily to address disease-imposed impairments. Nutritional programs designed for general health (e.g., the prevention of heart disease and certain forms of cancer) go beyond traditional dietary measures that target specific MS-related problems such as constipation and urinary infections. Practices such as yoga, meditation, mindfulness exercises, and tai chi also fall within the wellness concept. Stephanie comments on her experiences, focusing on wellness behaviors:

> *I learned to practice breathing exercises and meditation when I have a stressful day. Even when waiting in a line I can make my body relax for a few minutes. I also am careful about having a healthy diet. After school I either spend a half hour in the pool or take a walk if the weather is good. I think I have learned to enjoy life and pay attention to things that were not as important to me than before I was diagnosed with MS.*

In following a wellness approach, you can improve your general health and sense of wellness. MS may still cause symptoms and problems, but these are better managed by people who are physically and mentally stronger.

Some people fall guilty if they practice a healthy life style and still experience an attack of MS, feeling they should have tried harder, not missed that exercise session, or fallen off their diet. It is important to take responsibility for ways to keep yourself healthy but you are not responsible for the natural events that occur in the disease. Assuming this kind of personal responsibility for disease progression is both harmful and self-defeating. Your energy—emotional and otherwise—is better channeled into pursuing wellness, always recognizing that the goal is an overall improvement in general health rather than control of the disease process.

People who struggle to control their MS sometimes feel that they are losing the battle or "giving up" if they begin to use an assistive device. These devices actually extend your abilities by conserving energy, promoting safety, and reducing effort. For example, those who fatigue easily or struggle to be ambulatory with a cane or crutches will find that their activities become severely limited. All their energy is used simply to get from one place to another, leaving little or no effort to do or enjoy whatever activity had been planned. Struggling to get to the supermarket may mean that there is no energy left to shop. People with MS should use whatever techniques, tools, or devices are available to maximize and extend their activities and opportunities. Someone who is comfortable walking for short distances may choose to use a motorized scooter on a trip to an amusement park, shopping mall, or museum. A worker in a large office who normally uses a cane might also choose to use a scooter to conserve energy and enhance productivity. The effective use of assistive devices is an important extension of the wellness philosophy. They should be seen as a means of maintaining a full, productive, and enjoyable life rather than as symbols of defeat.

Children with MS

Although MS is considered an adult disease, it is estimated that there are between 10,000 and 20,000 children and teens with MS, or pre-MS symptoms, in the United States. This relatively uncommon situation presents special challenges to the family.

Establishing the diagnosis of MS in a child or teen can be fraught with even more difficulty than with an adult. The child is generally seen by a pediatric neurologist, who may not be accustomed to seeing this disease in children. In addition, there are non-MS conditions in children that make it difficult to sort out. As a result, months or years may go by before a diagnosis is established. Once a diagnosis of MS is made, issues for the child and family are also different. Parents worry about how they might have contributed to this diagnosis (not at all), and about the future of their child with a chronic disease, who will most likely outlive them. There is also the concern about normal childhood and teenage development and milestones. How will peers react, what about educational goals, and what will be the impact on critical social relationships?

The U.S. National Multiple Sclerosis Society has established six regional "Pediatric MS Centers of Excellence" that provide services unique to this population, and there are MS centers that address children's needs across Canada as well. Patients are assessed by a team who know the issues related to MS in younger people. In recent years there had been a lot of research on children with MS so it is not an unusual situation for the staff in MS centers. Rehabilitation, psychosocial, and other professional services are available through each of these centers, as well as care coordination.

Perhaps one of the most important areas for these children/teens is intervention with school personnel. Whether care is sought from one these centers or elsewhere, contact with the school is often critical. Most children with MS can and should continue with their normal schooling. The Society's six pediatric MS centers have staff to facilitate this, and the National Multiple Sclerosis Society chapters can provide additional help.

Also, the National Multiple Sclerosis Society and the Multiple Sclerosis Society of Canada have a multifaceted program to support families in this situation, which includes information, networking with other families, and telephone counseling.

Cultural Sensitivity

Disease is regarded differently in different cultures, so this may cause people with MS to experience different attitudes. Some cultures regard disease as a biological issue, but others may feel it is a weakness, or one's own fault, or due to a curse, or because of bad actions or sin. How others regard MS can profoundly affect how a person experiences the disease. Changing cultural beliefs is very difficult but patients, caregivers, and health professionals should be aware of how this can impact the lives of people with MS. It also can impact therapy, as the attitudes of different cultures to disease is reflected in their views on treatments as well.

Parting Thoughts

Amy relates her personal philosophy:

> If I had never had MS, I would never have traveled the way I did. I took a year off after I was diagnosed and traveled all around Europe. I decided I was going to do things while I could because I didn't know when something might be taken away from me. And I think one thing I've learned from MS is to do the things I can. It's a lesson for everyone. We should all live each day to the fullest, because we never know when something might happen to take it away.

Jim relates what gets him through:

> I would say that I have a lot of support from my family and friends. That probably helped me through. I had quite a few conversations, talks,

heart-to-heart discussions with different people, and that helped me quite a bit. Also, I'm somewhat religious and that helped.

Mary speaks about giving up denial:

I have this disease, I have done nothing to deserve it, and there is nothing I can do about having it. I just have to begin to take each day, one at a time, do my best, and accept whatever comes. The sheer honesty of admitting that I have an illness is a great weight off my mind. I am more attentive to details in my life, and more willing to do what my body tells me to do, instead of fighting against it. I have found a new calm I had not known before.

A religious or spiritual orientation has been linked with successful coping in a number of studies. It seems that religion helps some people find meaning in their illness, or at least put it into a meaningful context. Amy also refers to spirituality, as well as her own personal characteristics, as a support:

Since I grew up in a single parent household, I always had to draw on my own resources. So I worked really hard on that—and on my own sense of spirituality. I just had to—I've always depended on myself. I've always demanded a lot from myself and I guess I just drew it from within.

Amy refers to a key aspect of the coping process—a person's inner strengths. With an adult-onset disease, coping strategies have already been tested in other areas, creating a base on which to build. These strengths surface as the sense of crisis recedes. Amy has more advice for dealing with MS and with life in general.

Another thing is to laugh—to have a sense of humor. Don't take things so seriously. If you don't have a sense of humor, it's all for naught, you know. Life is too short. It can just really drag you down if you let it—you can't let that happen. Just try to take things one day at a time. One day at a time and "slow is fast enough," you don't really have to be in that much of a hurry. Take your time and take it easy and don't be afraid to ask for help.

When you have MS, hope is so important. Hope is justified. When we look at the history of MS in the early years in Chapter 1, and then look at the rapid changes occurring now in research, in the understanding of the disease, and in the remarkable development of increasingly effective MS drugs in the last few decades, we can see a positive future ahead.

CHAPTER 8

Employment Issues and Multiple Sclerosis

Many of us spend the majority of our waking hours at work and have a serious personal investment in and commitment to employment-related activities. Sometimes our self-image and identity are closely tied to our occupation or professional status. One of the first questions asked when getting to know someone is, "What kind of work do you do?" From a practical perspective, our income allows us to purchase goods and services to maintain our lifestyle and plan for the future. Work that is not associated with direct financial remuneration—such as parenting, homemaking, and volunteer activities—also contributes to our definition of self. These activities, however, *will* have a financial impact if they must be replaced by the paid work of others. Given all of these factors, it is not surprising that anything that potentially threatens the ability to continue employment or other productive and rewarding activity generates concern and anxiety. A diagnosis of MS certainly presents this kind of distressing situation.

The good news is that most people who discover that they have MS can and should continue working. The drugs approved for treatment of MS may help you to continue your employment status, although this factor has not been systematically studied.

Exacerbations may interfere with your usual work activities, but these episodes usually occur only on the average of about one a year or less in the early years of the relapsing-remitting form of the disease and decrease as time goes on. We see fewer relapses with earlier treatment with approved MS drugs. Progressive MS may require some changes in work activity, but disease limitations usually appear at a slow enough pace to allow for necessary modifications. It is important to be open with your employer about changes or adaptations you need in the work environment or routine that will allow you to continue to be fully productive. Employers already have made changes that are linked to prevention of disability, such as ergonomic desk chairs and hands-free headsets for the telephone. When put in this context, it likely will be easier for your employer to understand the benefit to productivity and the win-win situation for both of you.

When you receive a diagnosis of MS you may need to assess how this could affect your employment if symptoms occur. Usually for many years, people with MS carry on with their activities and employment as they are doing well, especially on treatment. Even attacks of MS symptoms are usually short in duration and with a good outcome in the early years. If symptoms remain, some adaptation at work may be necessary.

These factors are mentioned only to indicate that some adjustments may be needed in the workplace but are usually successful, and most people at work are understanding and supportive. If you have questions, discuss the situation with your employer or other staff members. Speak with others who have successfully managed MS and/or with a counselor who is experienced in helping people with MS think through the important issues related to employment.

Myths About MS

A number of myths or false beliefs make adjustment to MS more difficult. These misconceptions are held not only by a segment of the general public but also by an alarming number of health professionals who do not have extensive experience with MS and/or are unfamiliar with the professional literature. Some of them have a direct impact on the work experience. They include:

- ***Stress.*** At various points in the history of MS, stress was thought to worsen the disease and escalate the disease process. Scientific studies have examined this issue in detail, and results remain unclear about the role of stress in both the onset and the progression of MS. Advice to quit working, get help to care for children, and curtail volunteer activities is misguided if it is based only on the diagnosis of MS. Specific symptoms may have an impact, but they need to be evaluated individually and carefully because problems may be self-limited or responsive to symptomatic therapy.

- ***Activity.*** It was formerly believed that physical activity was detrimental to people with MS. The directive was to "take it easy," stop all physical exercise, and rest as much as possible. Bed rest was the primary recommendation for this erratic and unpredictable disease. The major public figure to challenge this notion was Olympic ski medalist Jimmie Heuga, who could not accept a life of inactivity. We now know that Jimmie was right and that activity and exercise are actually beneficial to the well-being of people with MS. It follows that work-related activity should not be curtailed unless dictated by specific, long-standing symptoms that have not responded to therapy.

- ***Incapacitation.*** Before MS was routinely recognized in its early stages and in mild cases, the common belief was that it would inevitably, and usually quickly, lead to serious disability that would interfere with the ability to perform daily activities, including employment. This is not true—most people with MS can often remain active and involved for many years.

Disclosure

The decision to communicate—or not to communicate—the diagnosis of MS in the workplace is complex and important and deserves careful consideration. Disclosure when interviewing for a new job poses different issues from disclosure when you already have an established position.

It is important to be aware of both legal and practical considerations whether you are seeking a new job or maintaining a current one. In the United States, people with disabilities are protected by the Americans with Disabilities Act (ADA), which became law in 1990. The definition of "disability" is complex, but may encompass MS regardless of whether symptoms are present. This is due to the possible perception of a disability. The employment section of the ADA states that individuals with disabilities who are covered under this law (a) have a mental or physical impairment that substantially limits one or more major life activities; (b) have a history of such an impairment; or (c) are perceived as having such an impairment. A diagnosis of MS carries such a possible preconception since an employer could potentially discriminate based on the association of MS with disability. The ADA prohibits employers from asking about or considering a diagnosis or general limitations in hiring and promotion decisions and only allows questions about ability to perform key components of the job. The ADA does offer the individual the option to request reasonable accommodations in order to perform those essential functions of your job. The challenge is that in order to tap into these protections under law, you would need to disclose that you have a disability and that it does affect one or more major life activities and that the accommodations you are requesting will assist you in effectively and efficiently completing the essential functions of your job. Determining who is the best person to disclose to, the best time to disclose, deciding what to say, and relating disclosure to accommodations are key things to be thinking about. It is important to identify the essential or key elements of your job because non-essential functions may potentially be delegated to or traded with other employees.

In a similar manner, Canadians are protected by the Employment Equity Act (Bill C-64) passed in 1995, which replaces the previous antidiscrimination legislation. This legislation seeks to eliminate employment barriers experienced by women, aboriginals, and visible minorities, as well as people with disabilities. Among the areas of concern that prompted this employment legislation was the severe underrepresentation in the workplace of people with disabilities.

Over time this has begun to change. Both the private and public sectors are covered by Bill C-64. The Act makes use of the Canadian Human Rights Tribunal (called the Employment Equity Review Tribunal when hearing employment equity cases). It also confirms the mandate for Human Resources Development of Canada to conduct research, provide labor market data, and administer programs to recognize outstanding achievement in employment equity. Both appeal procedures and enforcement measures are addressed.

In addition to legal considerations, people with MS are often concerned about health insurance, life insurance, and disability insurance. A prospective or current employee needs to explore policies relative to diagnosis of a chronic disease or occurrence of disability. "Preexisting condition" clauses must be carefully investigated, as well as "caps" (lifetime limits on expenditures for a particular condition or for an individual's total medical expenses) and related categories that potentially limit the availability of medical and health services because of MS or another chronic condition. These factors may or may not be disclosure related, depending on prior documentation of diagnosis and extent of information required for ongoing insurance coverage (see Chapter 9: "Financial and Life Planning").

The noninsurance, nonlegal aspects of working with MS often are more difficult to assess and address. Such considerations include anticipated employer and fellow employee support or lack of support, possible growth freeze if limitations are perceived by the employer, and personal emotional investment in efforts to acknowledge or deny issues related to MS. Colleagues, including supervisors, often rally to support a fellow worker with a health problem. In the case of MS, fund-raising teams have sometimes been created to support the individual who has been diagnosed through National Multiple Sclerosis Society events such as the "Walk" and "Bike Tour." Disclosure relieves the stress of covering up real needs and concerns and mobilizes team spirit and support.

You also need to disclose in order to request necessary accommodations. An accommodation may involve a change in scheduling, a parking space closer to the building entrance, or an office closer to the bathroom. Occasionally, equipment or a structural change such as a ramp may be needed. This is less often the case but usually is accomplished with minimal effort and cost when dealt with directly when the need is first identified. Many employers will permit and make it possible for you to work from home one or two days a week, an accommodation particularly helpful to someone bothered by fatigue.

An employer is required to make arrangements to help an employee perform "essential job functions." These accommodations must be "reasonable" in that they must be affordable and must not impose undue hardship on the employer.

There also are compelling reasons not to disclose: subtle or not so subtle pressure to resign, to accept lesser job responsibilities, or not to apply for promotion or expanded responsibilities. People have reported a "dead-end" feeling if a supervisor has clearly communicated lack of support for further advancement.

Resources

You probably do not need this information now and may never need it. However, you should be aware that such information exists at the time of diagnosis so that you can obtain appropriate assistance at the first sign of difficulty and avoid larger problems altogether.

Modest effort early on can prevent serious situations later and support your smooth career development.

Literature is available from the National Multiple Sclerosis Society in the United States (1-800-FIGHT-MS, www.-national mssociety.org) and the Multiple Sclerosis Society of Canada (NMSS; 416-922-6065, www.mssociety.ca/). Several publications are particularly helpful: *ADA and People with MS* by Cooper, Law, and Sarnoff, which is available as a download from the NMSS, details your protection under law in an easy-to-read style. Another downloadable brochure *The Win-Win Approach to Reasonable Accommodations* by Roessler and Rumrill, provides a practical guide to obtaining workplace accommodations and covers employment protections under the ADA and disclosure issues. You can also find *Should I Work? Information for Employees*, which gives a general overview of employment issues that might concern people newly diagnosed with MS, *Information for Employers*, and *A Place in the Workforce*, on the NMSS's site.

Every state has a vocational rehabilitation office; the phone number can be obtained through the telephone directory or information assistance, or online at www.jan.wvu.edu/sbses/-vocrehab .htm. If you look in the blue government pages of the telephone book under "State Government," this agency may be listed under one of the following headings:

- Department of Vocational Rehabilitation
- Department of Rehabilitation
- Department of Human Services
- Department of Social Services
- Department of Social and Rehabilitation Services
- Office of Vocational Rehabilitation

Each chapter of the National Multiple Sclerosis Society has a designated person who can address common employment issues. This "employment advisor" may be a trained chapter staff or volunteer in the community who is familiar with employment concerns of people with MS. This person will be able to address your questions and refer you to other employment resources and agencies.

In 2005, the National Multiple Sclerosis Society created the Career Crossroads: Employment and MS program. This program comprises a workbook and video/DVD that addresses common employment issues including disclosure, accommodation strategies, legal rights and responsibilities (ADA, FMLA), insurance issues (HIPAA, COBRA), and resources. Chapters may offer this training periodically, and the format may vary from chapter-to-chapter.

Some important resources include:

- Job Accommodation Network (JAN):

  1-800-526-7234, www.jan.wvu.edu

- JAN ADA Information Line:

  1-800-ADA-WORK (1-800-232-9675)

- ADA&IT Technical Assistance Centers:

  1-800-949-4232, www.adata.org

- Equal Employment Opportunity Commission (EEOC):

  1-800-669-4000, 1-800-669-6820 (TDD), www.eeoc.gov

- U.S. Department of Justice ADA Information Line:

  1-800-514-0301, www.ada.gov

The U.S. and Canadian MS societies have a general program for people recently diagnosed with MS called "Knowledge is Power," which can be accessed by calling 1-800-FIGHT-MS in the United States (www.nationalmssociety.org) and 416-922-6065 in Canada (www.mssociety.ca). Society chapters also have periodic educational programs for people recently diagnosed with MS and their families and include issues relative to employment. Some Society chapters have job retraining programs for people who need to make career changes in order to be able to continue working.

CHAPTER 9

Financial and Life Planning[1]

O ne part of dealing with MS is managing your money and plan-ning wisely for the future. Just as your MS symptoms are not exactly like someone else's symptoms, your financial situation also is unique. Now more than ever, you will need to take a clear look at your income, assets, debts, benefits, and other resources. This is something that you and your partner or family will probably need to do together.

At first glance, getting a good handle on your finances may seem overwhelming. If you give yourself some time and have a little patience, however, you can accomplish this step.

When I was first diagnosed with MS, I asked "Am I going to die?" The doctor said that, yes, someday I would die—but not from MS. That was more than 30 years ago. Since then, I've had my ups and downs, but I'm

---

[1] Modified with permission from *Adapting: Financial Planning for a Life with Multiple Sclerosis* pro-duced by the National Endowment for Financial Education.

still around, I still love life, and I've always managed to find a way to pay
for the things I need.

—Leslie, diagnosed in 1980

Getting Organized

An important first step is to gather the following materials. It is helpful to make copies and put them in labeled file folders in one location
that you can get to easily.

- Birth certificate
- Checking and savings account information
- Durable power of attorney document (establish one if you do
  not have one)
- Employee benefits information
- Insurance policies (life, health, disability, and long-term care)
- Investment account information
- Loans, including credit card statements
- Marriage certificate
- Military records
- Mortgage/deed of trust
- Social Security card
- Tax returns
- Titles (e.g., auto, house)
- Will

Professional Advisors

It is important to include the names and contact information of your
professional advisors with your financial file folders.

ADVISOR'S NAME	PHONE NUMBER
Accountant/tax preparer	
Financial planner	
Insurance agent	
Lawyer	
Others	

Taking a Financial Inventory

Review your MS symptoms to see if any of them may lead to additional expenses. For example, you may need to pay for regular massages to lessen muscle stiffness, or buy an air conditioner to keep your home cool because of sensitivity to heat. The spending plan worksheet (see the worksheet in the section "Developing a Spending Plan") also can help you estimate your monthly income and expenses.

Next, write down an estimated value of everything you own and the dollar amount of your debts. You'll want this information as you plan for future expenses or apply for any benefits that are based on financial need. As you do this estimate, take into consideration the Internal Revenue Service's definitions of value (go to www.irs.gov) and consider obtaining a professional appraisal of valuable assets, such as your home, artwork, jewelry, or other collectibles. Your accountant or other financial advisor can guide you.

Using a Health-Expense Spreadsheet

Another step you or a loved one can take is to create a health-expense spreadsheet, which should list items such as:

- Dates of doctor visits, hospital stays, or other treatments
- Charges for medical services, prescriptions, and medical supplies
- Portions of expenses covered by a health care plan

- Amounts and dates that you paid for health care services and any remaining balances
- Dates any deductibles were met, if applicable

Software programs can help you create a spreadsheet and will even do the math for you. If you do not own a computer, you can create a spreadsheet in a notebook or use the one provided in the section "Reviewing Your Health-Care Plan." Remember to keep copies of your supporting paperwork: doctor bills, health insurance statements, canceled checks, and bank statements in labeled file folders.

Realize that mistakes can happen when medical claims are processed. Even though these mistakes usually are unintentional, they can be costly. Check with your health care plan to see if it will share savings resulting from any errors you find in medical bills. Take careful notes while in the hospital or receiving treatment, and check the bill against your notes.

If you find possible billing errors, first try to resolve them with the doctor's or hospital's billing office. Next, get in touch with your health insurance company.

If the matter remains unresolved, contact your state's consumer protection office or insurance regulatory agency to file a complaint. Look in the blue pages of the phone book.

Reviewing Your Health Care Plan

As soon as possible, review your health care plan, so you will know what the plan will cover, what is excluded, and what your out-of-pocket expenses may be. Having this information will help you plan for anticipated medical expenses and strengthen an appeal on a claim if you believe it was denied incorrectly.

Health care plans can be difficult to read and understand, but there are people who can help you. Check the back of your health care card for phone numbers to call for information about your plan. If your health care plan is provided through an employer, someone in the employee benefits department may be able to answer your questions.

Health-Expense Spreadsheet

DATE OF SERVICE/ MEDICAL PURCHASE	CHARGES	AMOUNT/ DATE PAID BY HEALTH CARE PLAN	AMOUNT/ DATE PAID BY ME	DATE DEDUCTIBLE AND/OR COINSURANCE MET	DATE OUT-OF-POCKET LIMIT REACHED

When reviewing your plan, determine if it is a major-medical plan or a managed-care plan, such as a health maintenance organization (HMO), preferred provider organization (PPO), or point-of service plan (POS). Pay particular attention to information about copayments, coinsurance, deductibles, preexisting condition exclusion periods, lifetime maximums, and prescription drugs. These topics are discussed in the following sections.

Copayment

Most managed-care plans require you to pay a small amount, called the copayment or copay, each time you visit a health care provider within the plan's network. The amount of the copay may change annually. If your plan also has a deductible, the copay will not count toward it. Major-medical plans and some major medical-type benefits under managed-care plans do not have a copay.

Deductible

A deductible is the amount you must pay each year before a major-medical plan pays any expenses. For example, if your health care plan has a $500 deductible, you must pay the first $500 of covered medical costs before the plan begins to kick in. If the treatment is not covered by the plan, the cost for that treatment will not count toward the deductible. Managed-care plans, such as a PPO, HMO, or POS, may have a deductible if they permit care from out-of-network providers. Review your plan to determine which provisions apply to the provider you want to use.

Coinsurance

Coinsurance is the portion of a health care expense that you pay in addition to the deductible (when these provisions are part of your plan). A typical coinsurance provision says that after the deductible is paid, the health care plan pays 80 percent of covered charges for a treatment. You pay the other 20 percent. The percentage is your coinsurance amount. Plans vary as to the amount they expect you to pay.

Most plans have a "stop-loss," "breakpoint," or "out-of-pocket" limit. This is the maximum amount you will have to pay per person, or per family, each year. For example, an insurance company may have a stop-loss of $5,000. After you have paid $5,000 in deductible and coinsurance payments, the insurance company will pay 100 percent of covered expenses for the rest of the year. Check your plan for details.

Covered Expenses

Regardless of the amount charged by a provider, a plan will only cover certain treatments for certain amounts. Make sure you know what your plan considers a "covered expense," and if your health care provider will accept the plan's payment or will bill you for any amounts not covered by the plan.

Pre-existing Condition Exclusion Period

A pre-existing condition is a medical problem you had before you joined a health care plan. With a pre-existing condition, you may have to wait a period of time before the plan will cover that medical condition. This length of time could be three months, six months, or one year. As a rule, a group health plan cannot make you wait more than one year unless you did not enroll in the plan when first offered, in which case the waiting period may be as long as eighth months.

Under the Health Insurance Portability and Accountability Act (HIPAA), you will not have to meet a pre-existing condition exclusion period under a new plan if:

- You have had medical coverage for eighth months before changing to a new plan.
- You already have met a pre-existing condition exclusion period under a previous plan.
- You have not been without health care coverage for more than sixty-two days in the last twelve months.

Lifetime Maximums

Health care plans usually limit how much they will pay for health care through a "lifetime maximum benefit." When the limit is reached, the health care plan no longer pays for medical care. There also may be a limit for a single illness, injury, or condition, or an annual limit on certain medical services or equipment.

Prescription Drugs

Drugs for MS can be expensive. Plus, you likely will require other medications to manage symptoms. Even if your health care plan offers prescription drug coverage, you may have to pay part of the cost of these medications, so it is important to plan for this expense.

You can start by finding out whether the medications you need are covered by your health care plan. This information is available in the plan's "formulary," which is a list of drugs the plan will cover. Many health care plans cover some of the drugs that have been shown to modify the course of MS. What is on the formulary of your plan may make the selection of the immunotherapy for you.

If you are having difficulty paying for your medications, consider the following options:

- The companies that manufacture the major disease-modifying drugs may offer prescription drug assistance programs. Each program has its own qualifications. Begin by reading *Comparing the Disease-Modifying Drugs* (updated 2016), published by the National Multiple Sclerosis Society (www.nationalmssociety.org).

- Information about other prescription drug assistance programs for people with limited resources can be found at www.pharma.org. Several states also have prescription drug assistance programs.

- Talk to your doctor about prescribing a less expensive drug or helping you apply for a prescription drug assistance program.

- Shop for the best price and the best pharmacy. Compare local prices with mail order or online pharmacies, including delivery charges. If you decide to use a mail order or online pharmacy, choose one that requires a written prescription from your doctor. Be careful about using foreign pharmacies because of the importance of ensuring that the product you order is genuine, of the right strength, and uncontaminated.

- If you are a veteran, you may qualify for Department of Veterans Affairs (VA) health benefits, which include prescription drugs. You must enroll to receive benefits.

Family and Medical Leave Act

The Family and Medical Leave Act (FMLA) of 1993 requires employers with fifty or more workers, and all public/government employers, to provide up to twelve weeks of unpaid leave a year to eligible employees coping with certain family or medical situations. You can take the leave in small increments or all at once to care for yourself or an immediate family member, with the guarantee that you can keep your job and your health care benefits. Generally, the employer may decide whether FMLA time can be taken in installments.

To be eligible for FMLA leave, an employee must:

- Work for an employer that is covered by FMLA
- Have worked at the company for a total of twelve months
- Have worked at least 1,250 hours during the past twelve months

Employers may require employees to provide medical certification supporting the need for a leave due to a serious health condition affecting the employee or an immediate family member. In addition, when intermittent leave is needed for medical treatment, the employee must try to schedule the treatment so as not to unduly disrupt the employer's business.

Short-Term Disability Insurance

You may have disability insurance through your employer or on your own. The insurance might pay you a benefit if you experience either a short-term or a long-term disability that prevents you from working.

Keep in mind that even though an exacerbation is temporary, it can be disabling. Short-term disability insurance can help you through these times. With short-term disability insurance, which usually is available only through an employer, you can qualify for benefits within a few days or weeks of becoming disabled. The benefits can stop after a varied number of months, depending on the policy. Typically, you will be paid about 40 to 60 percent of your wages. You must report the benefit as taxable income if the employer paid the premiums for the insurance.

Job Changes and Health Care

One of the most important job benefits an employer can offer is a health care plan. Because MS is a lifelong condition, carefully consider the health benefits provided by an employer before accepting a position. Or, if you currently work for a company that does not offer a health care plan, you may want to look for a new job that has health care benefits.

In addition to COBRA, the HIPAA, also known as the Kennedy-Kassebaum Act, provides protection to individuals with a pre-existing condition when moving to a new health plan. HIPAA limits exclusions for pre-existing conditions and prohibits discrimination against employees and dependents based on their health status. This law guarantees that most workers with pre-existing conditions can move from their former group health plan to their new employer's plan without a break in coverage. For more information on HIPAA, go to www.dol.gov/pwba.

Don't ask to see the benefits package during the first interview, but when offered a job, ask to review the package before giving an answer. When reviewing the health care portion of the employer's benefits package, pay particular attention to the:

- Waiting period
- Pre-existing condition exclusion period
- Plan benefits and your costs

Taking Control of Finances

Developing a Spending Plan

The best way to know how much money you need to live on every month is to make a spending plan. Consider making several copies of the spending plan worksheets so you can use them throughout the year, or whenever your financial situation changes.

STEP 1: IDENTIFY YOUR INCOME

MONTHLY INCOME WORKSHEET	
SOURCES	**PER MONTH ($)**
After-tax wages	
Tips or bonuses	
Child support	
Alimony/maintenance payment(s)	
Unemployment compensation	
Social Security or Supplemental Security Income	
Retirement plan(s)	
Private disability insurance payments	
VA benefits	
Public assistance	
Food stamps	
Interest/investment income	
Other	
Total Income:	

STEP 2: LIST EXPENSES

MONTHLY EXPENSES WORKSHEET	
SOURCES	**PER MONTH ($)**
Mortgage or rent	
Utilities (heat, electricity, and water)	
Telephone, cell phone, Internet provider	
Groceries	
Transportation (bus fare, car payment, gas, repairs)	
Insurance (cost per month for car, home, health, and life insurance)	
Housekeeper/gardener, etc.	
Prescription drugs, medical supplies and equipment	
Treatments or therapies (massage, exercise classes, alternative treatments, supplements, etc.)	
Doctor/dentist bills	
Home adaptations or improvements	
Clothing/uniforms	
Child care/child support payments	
Alimony/maintenance payments	
Loan/credit card payments	
Entertainment (movies, eating out, etc.)	
Miscellaneous (e.g., classes, gifts, vacations, pet care)	
Donations	
Taxes	
Savings/retirement plan contributions	
Other	
Total Expenses:	

STEP 3: COMPARE INCOME AND EXPENSES

Write down your total monthly income (from Step 1).	$
Write down your total monthly expenses (from Step 2).	$
Subtract expenses from income and list amount here.	$

Looking at Investments

You may have money in a 401(K) or other retirement plan, or have other investments. It is a good idea to periodically review where your money is invested. The challenge is to find the right balance between the financial risk you can tolerate and the need for your money to grow.

If you currently are putting money into an employer-provided retirement plan, try to continue doing so. This is one of the best ways to save for your future—and you get special tax breaks. In addition, employers often match all or part of the money you save in the plan. Put at least enough money into the retirement plan to qualify for matching dollars from your employer.

Hiring a Financial Professional

If you decide to hire a financial planner to review your finances, ask the Multiple Sclerosis Society to refer you to professionals who have worked with people diagnosed with MS. The National Multiple Sclerosis Society in the United States has developed a partnership with the Society of Financial Professionals called the Financial Education Partners, which will provide volunteer professionals to meet one-on-one with people with MS. Be sure to call the Society at 1-800-FIGHT MS about this opportunity. In addition, the following organizations can provide names of financial planners near you:

- American Institute of Certified Public Accountants, Personal Financial Planning Division, www.cpapfs.org
- Financial Planning Association, www.fpanet.org
- National Association of Personal Financial Advisors, www.napfa.org
- Society of Financial Service Professionals, www.financialpro.org

Setting Aside Money for Unexpected Expenses

Many financial experts advise putting aside enough money to cover your bills for three to six months. This money can help if you lose your job or face other unexpected costs. Because you are dealing with a chronic disease, try to save enough money to cover six months of expenses.

The money you set aside for unexpected events should be placed in an account that you can get to easily. Consider the following options:

- *Savings account.* Savings accounts are easy to open and offer quick access to your money. While they pay only a small amount of interest, savings accounts at banks, savings and loans, and credits unions are safe investments.

- *Money market account.* You often need $1,000 to $10,000 to open a money market account. You may earn more interest on this type of account than with a savings account, but you may have limited access to it. In addition, depending on where you open a money market account, it may not be insured by the federal government. Be sure to ask.

- *Roth IRA.* Even though IRA stands for Individual Retirement Account, you can use a Roth IRA as a way to set money aside for emergencies. Unlike a regular IRA, you can withdraw the after-tax money you put into a Roth IRA without paying a penalty or taxes. However, generally you *cannot* withdraw any interest the account earns until age 59½ without paying a penalty. You are not taxed on any of the money you withdraw from a Roth IRA provided that you withdraw the money after age 59½, and the Roth IRA has been in existence for at least 5 years. However, if you become disabled, and distributions are made because of your disability, you do not have to meet the age 59½ rule for distributions of earnings to be income tax free.

To learn more about saving, investing, and personal finance, ask your librarian to recommend several good books. One great book on financial planning for all of those living with a chronic condition or disability is *Estate Planning for People with a Chronic Condition or*

Disability by Martin Shenkman, CPA, MBA, JD. This is not a book aimed only at people who have money; it will take you through living wills, determining how much life insurance your family needs and other financial matters. Or you can take a look at the following websites: Alliance for Investor Education, www.-investoreducation.org; American Savings Education Council, www.asec.org; Investment Company Institute, www.ici.org; or National Endowment for Financial Education, www.nefe.org.

CHAPTER 10

Research in Multiple Sclerosis: The Search for Answers and the Link to Treatments

R esearch in MS can help uncover fundamental knowledge of the disease's cause, the underlying mechanisms involved in the disease process, and its relationship to other disorders. This information is essential for developing safe and effective therapies. Indeed, the secret of acquiring effective ways to manage, prevent, and cure the disease will depend on a vigorous international research effort.

The first systematic studies of MS began in the mid-1800s by outlining the characteristics of the disease to separate it from other neurologic conditions. Physicians kept records on people with MS to show the various patterns of the disease, the pathological changes, and the response to treatments. It has evolved now, more than 150 years later, into a specialty area of basic and clinical research that incorporates virtually every discipline of modern medical science and biotechnology, ranging from clinical and community studies to the most up-to-date molecular laboratory techniques, genetic technologies, population studies, socioeconomics, psychology, and the application of randomized clinical trials to test new therapies.

Scientific research is a specialized discipline. Scientists are trained not only in their area of specialty research but also in the discipline and principles of scientific inquiry. Scientific research is driven by theories or hypotheses that then need to be challenged and tested using controlled laboratory or clinical techniques that have the greatest likelihood of providing meaningful answers. A *hypothesis* is a tentative assumption, usually developed through early observational study that can be proved or disproved by scientific investigation.

It has been said that the hardest part of science is asking the right question. The question has to be asked clearly so the hypothesis can then be stated in a way that also makes it clear how to test it.

Although there are many hypotheses in MS research, a great deal of investigation is currently directed at four major concepts about the disease and its cause (see Chapter 2):

1. It is a disorder resulting from an immune reaction in the central nervous system.
2. It occurs in genetically susceptible individuals
3. it is triggered by some other factor (infectious? environmental? other?).
4. It results in immune system–mediated inflammation and loss of the myelin and underlying nerve fibers of the brain and spinal cord, causing neurologic symptoms and the associated socioeconomic problems.

Research in Immunology—Uncovering the Root of the Disease

While MS is recognized as a disease of the brain, spinal cord, and optic nerves (the central nervous system), it is widely believed that

MS is caused by an immune system disorder that causes damage to central nervous system tissue. This disrupts the normal activity of the part of the central nervous system controlling movement, sensory perception, thinking, and emotional functioning.

The immune system of the body is complex and crucial to protecting us from attacks by a variety of threats such as bacteria, viruses, parasites, and other foreign substances that pose a threat. The immune system can identify that the foreign factors are different from our own body proteins, tissues, and cells. When something goes wrong and the immune system attacks its own tissue, it is called an auto-immune disease.

The immune system consists of the bone marrow, spleen, thymus, and lymph nodes. The bone marrow produces white blood cells, called leukocytes. The spleen contains many white blood cells that fight infection and foreign substances. The thymus gland is the place where T lymphocytes mature and help destroy infected or cancerous cells. The lymph nodes produce and store cells to fight infections. There are T and B lymphocytes that produce antibodies and help destroy infected or cancerous cells. Leukocytes are white blood cells that identify and eliminate infectious agents. There are also a host of regulatory substances that circulate in the blood called *cytokines* and *chemokines*, and many other key players.

Normal immune function protects the body from injury and disease caused by infectious agents—such as bacteria, viruses, and parasites—by mounting an attack against the "invaders" and clearing them from the body. Because our immune systems and our tissues and organs are all part and parcel of ourselves, our immune system recognizes our cells as "self." Thus, normally our individual body tissues are usually protected and not subject to attack by our own immune system. This "self-protection" is rooted in the identical genetic make-up of each person's immune system and other organs and tissues: The identical genetic background signals that the individual's tissues are a normal part of the body and should not be considered to be foreign invaders.

Sometimes, however, this innate protection goes awry and a person's own immune system begins to attack his or her own body tissues and organs as though they were foreign. Most scientists believe that this process may be the underlying cause of MS. The disease is the result of an abnormality in which a person's own immune system fails to distinguish foreign invaders from normal tissues in the body. As a consequence, the immune system attacks apparently normal body tissues as well as foreign invaders, resulting in inflammation and tissue damage that is often permanent.

Understanding immune function in the disease has helped to reveal important information on what happens in the disease and has allowed researchers to tailor new therapies that target specific aspects of the immune reaction. This is the basis of the disease modifying therapies (DMTs) available for MS patients today. We are now in a position to marshal this growing body of vital information about immune system function and dysfunction into the development of a new generation of therapies for MS.

Animal Model of MS: Experimental Allergic Encephalomyelitis (EAE)

In addition to human studies, immunological research in MS has been aided by animal models that have many of the immunological and pathological features of MS. It is *experimental allergic encephalomyelitis* (EAE), a laboratory-induced autoimmune disease of the brain and spinal cord in rats, mice, guinea pigs, and nonhuman primates. Studies of animal models for MS have greatly facilitated our understanding of basic immune system function and what goes wrong in autoimmune diseases. We recognize that EAE is not MS but studying the immune changes in EAE has been useful in understanding how the nervous system can be damaged by an immune reaction.

Because MS involves the immune system, physicians have used powerful drugs that modify immune function by decreasing the growth and proliferation of immune cells. Many such therapies that have been tested for MS—drugs such as cyclophosphamide and azathioprine and procedures such as total body or total lymphoid irradiation—have global or widespread immunosuppressive effects, potentially leaving a treated patient open to a variety of infections and complications. This complication has made these therapies of questionable value in terms of *risk versus benefit.* Even while recognizing that some of these agents might be able to help control the disease process, the risks of serious short-term complications and long-term risks such as malignancies, has limited their acceptance and use. Pinpointing the exact immune problems in MS has long been a goal of scientists. It is thought that such information could lead to highly specific therapies aimed at those immune system components involved in the disease, while leaving the rest of the immune system intact and functioning.

This search has been an important focus of research in recent years. This includes exploring what makes an immune system that is normally directed against outside invaders become misdirected against normal body tissues. Why the body mistakes "self" tissue for "foreign" invaders, and searching for the actual target of immune responses in the brain and spinal cord. Scientists are trying to determine the nature of T cells and antibodies that are primed to attack this target.

Another promising avenue of immunological research is directed at understanding how and why immune system cells move from the bloodstream into the central nervous system. This phenomenon, called "trafficking," may be one of the most important aspects of immune system problems in MS. Ordinarily, activated immune cells that could cause damage in the central nervous system are prevented from moving from the blood to the nervous system. In MS, the blood-brain barrier that keeps activated immune cells in the blood is breached and the potentially damaging cells enter the nervous system. Why is the blood-brain barrier breached in MS? How can the resulting movement of cells into the nervous system be stopped? Within recent years, a sufficient body of information has accumulated that points to the development of therapies that can block the blood-brain barrier breach and reduce or prevent immune cells from trafficking into the brain. Continuing work is needed to develop drugs that more effectively and safely reduce trafficking of immune cells into the central nervous system.

A difficulty in the MS research is the uncertainty about what specific antigens in myelin are being targeted in the immune reaction. One difficulty may be that there could be multiple myelin antigens involved. It is possible that different people may have different antigenic responses. To complicate things further, there tends to be a shifting in the immune responses. This means that specific T-cell treatments aimed at taking advantage of the originally proposed "restricted" immune responses in MS would not likely to be effective for a wide spectrum of patients with MS, and treatments effective at one time in the disease may not continue to be effective.

One relatively new focus in immunological research in MS has been on chemical messengers of the immune system called *cytokines* and *chemokines.* Cytokines and chemokines are produced by immune and other cells that regulate immune system activity. Many scientists believe that cytokines may be important "final pathways" involved in all immune responses—some cytokines encourage inflammation, which can be damaging in MS, and others suppress inflammation, which may be protective in MS. By manipulating cytokine activity so that pro-inflammatory responses are suppressed and anti-inflammatory responses are encouraged, it may not be necessary to understand specific immune cell responses in MS to combat the disease. And a second group of immune messengers, chemokines, sends important information signals throughout the body, helping to direct immune responses where they need to be most active. Controlling these chemical messengers may provide a kind of relatively non-specific treatment for MS.

Interferons, which are one type of cytokine, are an example of this dichotomy: Interferon beta has been shown to be anti-inflammatory and has been beneficial for treating MS, while there is evidence that interferon gamma may make the disease worse, at least at certain stages of the disease. Enhancing the activity of interferon beta might be an effective treatment; suppressing gamma interferons at certain states of the disease might be successful as well. A number of approved therapies for MS provide interferon beta by injection.

Research is giving us a better understanding of the cytokine "networks" and chemokine signaling pathways that are involved in MS and we hope to learn how to block "bad" cytokines and chemokines and enhance the effects of "good" ones.

Much of what we know about immunology and autoimmunity, including the actions of cytokines and chemokines, is shared among different autoimmune diseases. However, even if such complex immune networks are understood in a different disease, the outcomes are not always predictable in MS. For example, an important cytokine called tumor necrosis factor alpha (TNFα) was found to be involved in nervous system tissue damage in animal models of MS and believed to be functioning abnormally in MS itself. Blocking the action of TNFα in animal studies prevented or improved disease. A similar phenomenon was seen in animal models of rheumatoid arthritis that resulted in successful clinical trials for an agent that blocks TNFα in that disease, which is now available to treat arthritis patients. It was disappointing to find in clinical trials in MS that such TNFα blockers actually worsened MS. As before, as informative as animal and other disease research may be for MS, it is not always possible to predict MS-specific results. This is why careful, stepwise research needs to be conducted. Controlling cytokine activity in MS, such as interleukin-2 (IL-2), which can foster harmful inflammatory activity in the brain in animal models and in MS, is a fruitful area for the development of monoclonal antibody that can block the activity of IL-2.

While most work in MS immunology has focused on the T-cell response, cytokines, and chemokines, antibodies produced by B cells are increasingly believed to be important in MS pathology as well, and some of the newest effective treatments are directed at reducing B cells. The recent focus on antibodies as an important part of the MS pathology has led to attempts to control antibody responses using agents that specifically block the immune B cells that produce them.

Hormones

Also important is research on the role of hormones in MS. It is well known that MS is three times as common in women as in men. And it is well known that pregnant women with MS tend to have stabilization or improvement of their disease in the second and third trimesters of pregnancy, when estrogen levels are high, only to experience a higher risk for a disease exacerbation in the first several months after delivery, when estrogen levels drop. Changes in estrogen levels during pregnancy are thought to help regulate immune function: The immune system is suppressed in pregnancy to prevent a "rejection" of the fetus, which is recognized as being foreign by the mother's immune system. Therefore, hormone regulation of immune responses in MS has been an important area of MS research in recent years. Estrogen can actually improve EAE, the animal model of MS; testosterone, a male sex hormone, can make the disease worse. Would hormone levels also help control MS in humans by regulating immune function? This is under study.

Genetic Research—Links to Susceptibility, Course, and Causation

Research on the genetic basis of MS has clarified some of the patterns of MS in families and populations. Population studies tell us that specific groups of people may be protected from MS and others may be more susceptible, with different rates of MS in different parts of the world (see Chapter 2). Moving beyond population studies, genetics research has become highly "molecular" in nature as scientists race to uncover genetic factors that underlie the disease and may help determine who is susceptible. The worldwide effort that led to the understanding of the human genome has helped us understand the genetic code that defines humans and was a major step in unraveling the complexities of diseases with genetic components. Whole genomic screens in MS have supported hypotheses about its autoimmune nature. They still have not explained the exact genetic basis of the disease. Genomic screen studies have now led to a focus on analysis of genetic haplotypes—blocks of genes that tend to be inherited together and that may be used for easier analysis of genetic factors in diseases like MS.

The possibility of specific gene therapies is no longer the stuff of science fiction, even though its application to human disease is in the early stages. The first attempts unfortunately were unsuccessful in disorders such as metabolic diseases and muscular dystrophy. There are very strict ethical and governmental restraints on gene therapy studies in humans. For gene therapy to become a potential treatment in a disease like MS, we need to understand completely the genetic factors that underlie the disease and devise ways to "correct" any defects that may be present. We are a long way from this goal and, given the nature of the disease, it may not be possible to achieve it at all.

A more immediate consequence of genetic research in MS may be the development of techniques to more readily determine susceptibility to MS in the general population and in families in which the disease already occurs. Genetic factors may even one day provide some clues to the prognosis for any individual with the disease, helping to predict the type of MS that a person will have and even its severity.

The genetic research has supported the belief that MS is autoimmune in nature. Immune function is under strict genetic control, and the genes of people with MS that control immune function are in some ways different from the immune system genes of healthy individuals. Among these are genes involved in helping the immune system determine which body tissues are its own and which substances are foreign—a bacterium or virus or even a transplanted liver or kidney from a genetically different donor. This ability to distinguish between self and foreign allows the immune system to mount an effective response against foreign substances but not against tissues or cells that are part of its own body. Genes controlling this recognition process are called human leukocyte antigens (HLA genes), histocompatibility genes, or major histocompatibility genes (MHC genes). Based on both early population studies in which HLA typing was done on blood samples and more recent results from highly molecular state-of-the-art whole genome screens of individuals with MS in the United States, Canada, and the United Kingdom, the HLA genes are, to date, the strongest link that we have to an MS genetic factor.

Genetic studies are helping us to know more about the immune nature of the disease, how much of the disease susceptibility may be related to genetic problems in immune system function, and how much of it may be related to other non-immunological factors or even to environmental or infectious factors.

An interesting recent genetic observation is a link between MS and vitamin D. It was shown that proteins activated by vitamin D in the body bind to a particular DNA sequence lying next to the DRB1-1501 variant associated with MS risk.

Microbiome – How Bacteria in the Gut Affect the Immune System

The microbiome is the population of bacteria in the small and large intestine of the digestive system, which has more cells than in the rest of the body. There is increasing information on how the balance of the bacteria in the gut is important to health, and how alteration can affect many diseases and affect the immune system. There is evidence that the microbiome is involved in cardiovascular disease, obesity, and inflammatory bowel disease. Early research suggests the microbiome in MS patients may be different from other people and further research will try to find out the details and what factors might alter it back to normal. We also know that factors of interest in MS such as vitamin D deficiency, smoking, and alcohol can affect the microbiome. There are promising studies in laboratory animals to show that demyelinating disease (EAE) similar to MS can be worsened or improved by altering the microbiome in various ways. There are studies underway to see how the microbiome may be involved in the disease and how therapeutic trials could be designed.

Infectious Disease Research—Clues to Triggers, Causes, and Possibly Treatments

Genes and the immune system are clearly involved with MS, but what event actually triggers the development of MS in people who are susceptible? For over a century it was suspected that an infection might be the trigger for MS, but it has been hard to prove and the evidence is incomplete.

Viral infections can cause human diseases with characteristics similar to those of MS, and these are usually one-time acute events. Certain viral diseases in laboratory animals also result in myelin damage like that seen in MS. For decades there has been very clear evidence that some viral infections, particularly upper respiratory tract viral infections, may set off acute exacerbations of MS in individuals who already have the disease. These observations, along with the knowledge that MS is more common in temperate regions and rare in tropical regions, have generated years of scientific hypotheses about infectious agents and MS. Some infectious diseases have a geographic pattern, as MS does, and it was noted many years ago that polio, when it was widespread, had a pattern not dissimilar to MS. There are many other infections common in temperate zones, but less common at the Equator, and vice versa.

Researchers have hunted for a specific identifiable virus related to MS, with the hope that this will result in a relatively simple explanation for the disease, and also with the hope that combating such a virus with a specific vaccination will result in a safe and effective preventive treatment or a specific virus-focused disease treatment. However, the search for *the* MS virus has been unfruitful. Several dozen common and uncommon viruses have been postulated to be related to MS based on either epidemiologic studies, the presence of higher levels of antibodies against a given virus in individuals with MS, or, more recently, evidence from very sophisticated polymerase chain reaction (PCR) analysis that can detect the "footprint" of a viral protein in body fluids and tissues even if the virus has been long eliminated by the immune system.

In most cases follow-up studies confirming the relationship of MS to a specific virus have not been convincing. Most such claims have been a result of inadequate experimental sampling or laboratory contamination. Nonetheless, there remains the possibility that infections may be related to MS.

In recent years, most of the focus has been on viruses that are very common in the general population—not necessarily isolated only in individuals with MS—such as human herpesvirus 6, which causes roseola in infants, and Epstein-Barr virus (EBV), which is known as the cause of infectious mononucleosis. Virtually everyone in the population has been exposed to these viruses, making it hard to assess a connection to MS.

A common bacterial infection has similarly been linked to MS. *Chlamydia pneumoniae*, the cause of "walking pneumonia," is an infectious agent to which most humans have been exposed. Reports have claimed an association with this bacterium in individuals with MS and have shown its presence in MS tissues. But many years of follow-up research have raised skepticism about the original reports, and a causal relationship between this bacterium and MS has not been proven.

How can common infectious agents be involved with MS when relatively few humans have the disease? Are these false leads and not really causes of MS? Are such agents simply associated with MS or are they "cofactors" that are required, but not in themselves sufficient, to cause the disease? If so, what else might be required for the disease to appear? This is where *genetic susceptibility* may have its impact: While a common infectious agent may be a trigger for MS, perhaps the disease will only occur in people who carry a genetic susceptibility to it. It is probable that both—a triggering agent and the "right" genetic background—are required and neither alone is sufficient for MS to develop.

This may be the case, but many investigators believe it is likely that no specific virus, bacterium, or other infectious agent will be found to be a cause of MS. Instead they are concentrating on research that explores how a susceptible person's immune system reacts to a variety of viral or other infections, or how immune function is tied to hormonal and other factors that might explain the initiation of the MS process. Studies from the mid-1990s to now, largely in laboratory animals, have helped to explain how an immune system that has lost its ability to distinguish self from non-self-tissue can be tricked by certain infectious agents into mounting an attack against its own myelin. The "trick" might be a very close similarity of molecular structure among some viruses, bacteria, and myelin itself—called *molecular mimicry* to reflect the similarity of molecular structure between some parts of myelin and some infectious agents. An effective and natural immune response mounted against a common infectious agent might result in a damaging cross-reaction with myelin itself if the molecular structure of the infectious agent mimics part of the molecular structure of myelin. This scenario of "mistaken identity" may explain much of the origin of MS and help to determine how the disease can be prevented from occurring in susceptible people.

Glial Cell Research—What Is Damaged? What Can Be Repaired?

The symptoms of MS are directly due to inflammation and breakdown of myelin and the cells that make myelin called *oligodendrocytes*. Most likely as a secondary (but still early) process, nerve fibers that are wrapped and insulated by myelin also are often damaged in MS. The biology of oligodendrocytes and other glial cells in the central nervous system is a vital and expanding area of research. This includes study of how oligodendrocytes develop and form myelin in early stages of life, how they are affected by immune system responses, how the nervous system responds when myelin is lost, how scars are formed when myelin is lost, and what the potential is for myelin regeneration and recovery.

Basic biochemical studies of myelin using increasingly sophisticated techniques have closely analyzed nervous system tissue in people with MS, and such studies are used to determine if there are any abnormalities in the myelin or oligodendrocytes that might make these tissues and cells vulnerable to immune system attack. Historically, biochemical and anatomic research have repeatedly demonstrated that myelin, or white matter, is "normal" in individuals with MS, suggesting that the autoimmune attack in MS is truly a question of immune cells not recognizing normal self-tissue.

However, by the mid-1990s, a new technology stemming from magnetic resonance imaging (MRI), called *magnetic resonance spectroscopy* (MRS), began to show that normal-appearing white matter (myelin) in the brains of people with MS may actually have subtle abnormalities. It is not clear if these subtle imaging signals truly reveal myelin tissues or oligodendrocytic cells that are potentially vulnerable to immune attack or whether such signals are a result of a very early, previously undetected disease process. Cause and effect here, as elsewhere in biomedical research, is difficult to sort out. But such studies show not only the power of newer technologies but also the need to constantly reassess scientific beliefs and facts. Subsequently there have been pathological studies that also show that there is evidence of abnormal change in the areas that initially looked normal. We still need to consider, therefore, that there may be inherent abnormalities in white matter and myelin in individuals who develop MS and that the immune response is directed against this abnormal tissue. Or the disease is more widespread than suspected from clinical findings and MRI.

Regeneration and Repair

Early on it was not recognized that myelin in the central nervous system could be regenerated after it was damaged. In the 1980s it was found that there was a degree of new myelin development in individuals whose brains showed extensive immune system damage and scarring due to MS. This myelin regeneration was insufficient to overcome the devastation caused by the disease, but it provided new hope that myelin could be more effectively repaired. It is likely that regeneration is very active early in the disease but repeated damage over time makes it harder to repair the myelin.

Knowing that damaged central nervous system oligodendrocytes can regenerate and form new myelin, many laboratories have focused on ways to enhance myelin growth and development in animals and in humans. In most cases of MS, particularly early cases, when myelin insulation around nerve fibers is damaged or lost, the central axon remains intact and can continue to function when myelin is restored, even though the new myelin is thinner than before. This is why we see recovery after an attack of MS.

Scientists are pursuing many experimental approaches to meet this challenge. These include identifying the early-stage myelin-making cells in the nervous system, called *oligodendrocyte progenitors*, that are capable, even in adults, of forming new tissue after immune system damage; using "growth factors" to stimulate myelin regeneration; taking advantage of chemical and physical signals that flow between myelin and nerve fibers to stimulate more rapid and efficient myelin growth and nerve regeneration; modulating immune system functions by blocking special immunoglobulins and antibodies that may be inhibiting myelin growth; and transplanting myelin-making cells from healthy donors or from healthy parts of a person's own nervous system to diseased or damaged nervous system sites.

Stem Cell Research

Concepts of transplantation of myelin-making cells or of nerve cells by necessity involve research related to stem cells. Many of the ethical and religious concerns were solved when it became possible to develop stem cells from the tissues of the person who would in turn receive the stem cells. A key problem in cell or tissue transplantation is the issue of immune system rejection of the transplanted cells and tissues, based on a lack of genetic compatibility of the donor with the recipient, so this is overcome by using the person's own stem cells. So, the potential of therapeutic cloning of cells from the patient is a major advance. This research is opening doors to future ways to treat MS.

There are a number of studies that use bone marrow depletion by drugs and then replacement with the patient's own stem cells. This a difficult and complex therapy for a patient, but most of the cases have been advancing MS that failed on other therapies. The results have been very dramatic and positive.

To date, studies focused on myelin and nerve regeneration and replacement in MS (not using bone marrow suppression) have been largely limited to laboratory experimentation. Studies using certain immunoglobulins to suppress a theorized immunologic inhibition of myelin growth have been done in humans with MS, with mixed results; more work is planned. One small study that attempted to show re-myelination by transplanting peripheral nervous system glial cells into the brains of individuals with MS did not meet with success. But these are the first steps, and over time, more such efforts will be made, and eventually one or more of the cutting-edge techniques may prove to be successful. All of this research provides hope that myelin regrowth and functional recovery for individuals with MS may be possible in the future.

However, no matter what the potential for myelin and nerve fiber regeneration and growth, it is vital to emphasize two key problems related to MS: (a) the continuing immunological reaction, if unchecked, will tend to overcome efforts for regeneration; and (b) for some individuals, especially those with advanced MS, long-standing nerve fiber damage is likely to be a major component of their disability. Even if myelin can be repaired for such individuals, if the nerve fiber, the axon, is damaged, it is unlikely that conduction can be restored. Thus, research focusing on myelin and nerve regeneration must move hand-in-hand with efforts to stop the underlying immune system process—both to prevent patients from becoming seriously disabled in the first place and to hold in check immune system activity that will simply continue to damage any repaired cells and tissues. It is also another reason to treat MS early to take advantage of current therapies to reduce the activity of the disease.

Clinical Research—Treating the Whole Patient

Clinical research directly involves individuals who have MS—not test tubes, not laboratory animals, but individuals living with a chronic disabling disease who experience symptoms, impediments to activities of daily living, and who have to live with consequent impacts on employment, family life, and social interactions. All MS research, no matter how fundamental, is aimed at finding treatments and a cure and at improving the quality of life for people living with MS. Studies in basic immunology, virology, and glial biology, in laboratory test tubes or in animal models of MS, all become applied in the clinic to help us translate such fundamental disease information into studies of people with MS. Clinical trials (see Chapter 11) focus on testing the safety and efficacy of new drugs and agents developed to treat MS and its symptoms (Figure 1).

Also important is the refinement and development of new techniques for reaching a diagnosis. Such techniques can be used to follow disease progress, particularly the relatively new imaging techniques based on magnetic resonance technology that allow direct observation of lesions in the brain and spinal cord (MRI and related technologies). New developments in analysis of MRI, blood, and cerebrospinal fluid also have importance in diagnosis, in tracking disease change over time, and in monitoring the results of experimental clinical studies. These technologies played a role in recent refinements of criteria used to diagnosis MS. In particular, the value of imaging and how it should be used has been codified into new MS diagnostic criteria through the widely used McDonald MS Diagnostic Criteria first put forth in 2001 and since refined in 2005 and 2010 (see Chapter 1).

Figure 1.　The spectrum of MS research.

Basic Research →	Clinical Research →	Patient Management, Care and Rehabilitation → Research	Health Care Delivery and Policy Research
aims to	aims to	aims to	aims to
Understand Biologic → Mechanisms	Apply Basic Understanding → to Treat, Prevent, Cure	Improve Symptoms and Quality of Life →	Optimize Delivery of Care and Guide Public Policy

While new treatments are being developed to help reduce the symptoms and progression of MS, helping individuals and their families cope with the disease, obtain the best possible medical care, and function at the highest possible level in society are essential aspects of research in the areas of psychosocial studies as well as health care delivery and policy research.

Understanding the psychologic and emotional aspects of MS has become a major focus of research in recent years. We realize that the brain pathology of the disease creates problems in cognitive and emotional function. Increased information in these areas is leading to new techniques to help with coping and rehabilitation, as well as interventions that can be applied in a clinical setting.

Although not limited to MS, the problems of access to care and services for people with chronic disease are increasingly unwieldy and are becoming the focus of high-quality health care delivery and policy research. Data gathered from such studies have a direct impact on altering public perception of chronic disease and on changing for the better legislative policy, entitlement programs, and societal policy for all people with disabilities.

Current research in MS is broad based and comprehensive. Funding for this research traditionally has come from governmental agencies, MS societies in many countries around the world, and, more recently, pharmaceutical and biotechnology companies. The results have increased understanding of the disease, provided new and specific therapies, and significantly enhanced the quality of life for people with MS. Basic and applied research are needed more than ever before to close the gaps in our knowledge of MS and move us closer to full treatment, prevention, and cure.

CHAPTER 11

Searching for Treatments: The "Ins" and "Outs" of Clinical Trials

Biomedical research in MS is intended to better understand the underlying mechanism and cause of the disease, which will lead to safe and effective therapy. The process is to explore research areas of immunology, virology, genetics, and neurophysiology to develop more focused therapies to benefit people with MS. When the research develops a potentially helpful drug, device or other therapy, the way to assess the benefit and safety of the therapy is by a *randomized, double-blinded clinical trial (RCT)*.

The Randomized Clinical Trial

The RCT is designed to avoid bias in the assessment of results of treatment. Many things may appear to work when the results are no better than chance, and are biased by the desire to see a positive result.

In a RCT the drug to be studied is given to a large group of patients who are from a randomized population of MS patients and compared to a matched group who are reasonably the same so the results can be compared. One group is given the drug and the other an identical appearing placebo (or a comparable drug to study one against the other). The physicians, nurses and patients don't know who has the active drug and the inactive drug (blinded to the therapy). The only group who knows and oversees the trial as it goes along is a safety committee that makes sure nothing untoward happens. The RCT is the gold standard for the study of a drug.

It may seem an easy task to test a promising new drug, but consider the steps. First there has to be some solid scientific basis for considering a clinical trial of a drug and this may have come only after years of basic research. Then it is a long process to design the study, and determine how many patients have to be studied, for how long, to obtain a convincing statistical result. Then it has to go through a rigorous ethical review by an ethics committee. Then, if the study is not funded by the company who developed the drug, it will have to be presented to a funding agency in hopes that it will receive support. The application process may take a year or more. When funded, the recruitment of hundreds of patients may take one or two years, and the duration each patient must be followed is usually many years. After the trial is ended and all patients have arrived at the end of their treatment phase, it would take a year to collect all the data, do the statistical analysis, submit the results to a major medical meeting, and submit the finished research paper to a journal.

It would be nice if this could be faster, and many efforts are being made, with assurance that the quality of the results would not be lessened, but it still is a long procedure in order to get it right. The interferons were discovered in the 1970s but approved for therapy of MS after trials in the 1990s. It was twenty-five years from the discovery of glatiramer acetate to having it approved by the Food and Drug Administration for MS therapy. New technologies such as MRI are allowing us to do some trials more quickly but it still takes time and costs are often in the $15 million to $30 million range. We should also recognize that all this time, patient involvement, expense, and hope could end in failure, because the drug was ineffective, or had too many risks, or good but no better than available therapies. Poorly done clinical trials that result in misleading conclusions are wasteful at best and potentially dangerous for the intended population needing the treatment if they provide erroneous conclusions.

The Special Problems of MS Trials

Placebo Effects

Almost every drug used in every disease has a placebo effect, a feeling or sense of improvement that is due to the mind's positive perception of a result, unrelated to the effect of the treatment. And in the case of a placebo, which has no effect, the placebo effect again is due to the mind's perception, and the feelings are real, not imaginary. For example, in a study patients were told the drug (actually an inert placebo) was a stimulant and the patients' had an increased heart rate, increased blood pressure, and more rapid reaction times, but when told it was a sleeping pill they had the opposite reaction. Some pain and headache studies have very high placebo effects. In all the trials of MS drugs that showed benefit, the placebo group had some positive results as well. What the study has to show is that the drug effect is greater than occurs with a placebo. Placebo effects are very complex, as a red pill has a greater effect as a stimulant, and a blue pill has a greater effect on sleep. Also taking two placebo pills has a greater effect than one. And being told the placebo pill is very expensive has a greater effect, as does putting it in a package that has a known trade name over a plain package.

People with MS generally are highly motivated to search for a treatment or cure for their disease and hope for benefit in any treatment. This positive motivation can actually interfere with the objective assessment of any drug or device. Working with a sympathetic physician who also strongly believes in the value of an experimental treatment can help to reinforce placebo effects and can give rise to false-positive outcomes in clinical trials.

Simply participating in a clinical trial can result in a person's sense of well-being and increased hope and excitement at the prospect that an experimental agent will have benefit. As we mentioned, the placebo effect is not imaginary. The positive psychologic factors can even affect immune system function, thus leading to a real change in immunology that could have a direct impact on this immune-mediated disease. The interaction between psychology, physiology, and disease outcomes in MS is not well understood, but when they occur, they can seem to cause disease improvement—usually temporary unfortunately, since the underlying disease process might be unaffected. Such placebo effects are particularly present when results of experimental treatment rely on self-reporting of symptoms or physical state by a treated patient rather than on the more rigorous objective assessment of performance by an examining physician or on objective laboratory findings. This was noted in clinical trials of CCSVI when a large number of patients said they felt improvement in symptoms, but there was no improvement and sometimes worsening in objective measurements of their MS.

While important and potentially useful, placebo effects must be carefully separated from a true therapeutic drug effect. Treatments are costly, often inconvenient, and usually have associated side effects. If the impact of a treatment is, in fact, no better than a placebo response, there is no reason to use the drug! So, any useful drug for MS must have an impact that is greater than the placebo effect.

The Natural Disease Variability of MS

The high degree of variability in MS makes the design of clinical trials difficult. The patients have different involvement, different courses, and because it is a life-long disease, the changes are usually slight in any year. In any individual, the disease may go through seemingly spontaneous remission and worsening that are unpredictable in occurrence, severity, and duration; no two individuals experience the same problems in the same ways. Spontaneous stabilization in previously progressive disease or a spontaneous remission of symptoms could easily be confused with a drug effect even if the drug is having no impact whatsoever.

Understanding the Predicted Drug Effect

New agents for MS are usually chosen for testing because their known or suspected mechanism of action bears some relation to what we know about the disease. For instance, because the disease is widely believed to have an immune system origin, most new agents being tested in MS work through modulating immune functions. However, drugs may have different effects on different MS disease types. Agents that may be predicted to alter the frequency or severity of acute attacks of MS may have no benefit on longer term progression of disease, which may be due more to tissue degeneration than to inflammation.

A trial is designed to study a defined outcome, so certain patients who fit that criteria are candidates, but not others. For instance, if the study is to see if a drug has an effect on acute attacks, only patients who are having a certain number of acute attacks each year would be included.

Finally, some drugs may seem to cause improvement but actually only have indirect effects on the MS disease process. This can be the case for agents aimed at treating symptoms of MS like spasticity, fatigue, or depression, in which improvement may be real, but only the symptom and not the underlying disease is affected. This does not make the intervention less valuable, but it is important to distinguish between symptom improvement and actual impact on the underlying disease pathology that might come from disease-modifying agents. Understanding the true effect of any drug on the disease process requires a detailed knowledge of the drug's action and careful clinical assessment of effects on the disease.

Availability of Safe and Useful Therapies

Since 1993 a total of fifteen drugs have been approved for the treatment of MS by the Food and Drug Administration and by other drug regulatory authorities in countries around the world. The list of approved drugs in each country may vary as each country has its own process to approve new drugs. The approval process requires convincing clinical trial data, which are examined in great detail.

The availability of treatments for some forms of MS actually complicates the search for new therapies, as placebo trials are less accepted now that many effective therapies are available. Increasingly the new agent must be tested against a known therapy. This has been specifically addressed in recent revisions of the Declaration of Helsinki, an international agreement that sets out guidelines for all human research. The Declaration states that it is an ethical obligation to provide "best available therapy" to all patients involved in research. It would be unethical to withhold known effective therapy, so trials in the future will mostly compare the experimental therapy with an accepted therapy rather than a placebo.

Beyond ethics, there are other issues involved in conducting placebo-controlled studies. Many patients don't want to enter a trial where they may receive a placebo rather than the study drug. This makes recruitment of patients difficult.

Comparison of New Treatments Against Available Therapies

New treatments that are being developed need to be at least as good as, but hopefully, better than those already available. One way to judge is to conduct a "head-to-head" clinical trial that can determine clinical superiority of one agent over the other. Superiority might be determined by showing increased efficacy of one agent compared to the other, but also by increased safety, increased ease of delivery or compliance, or all of these. For statistical reasons, and because trials are conducted differently, it is difficult to compare the results of two separate placebo-controlled trials of two different agents, each tested alone against placebo, and to say that one is better than the other. All studies have a different patient population, are done in different locations, and are done at different times, all of which make direct comparisons between outcomes of different trials done at different times impossible. Head-to-head studies are difficult and expensive but more and more trials will be by this method.

These and other problems associated with MS clinical trials can best be overcome by extremely rigorous experimental designs for the studies. The generally accepted methods of study are time consuming and expensive, and needed innovation is hard to come by, but such rigorous trial designs hold the best chance of obtaining a clear-cut answer about the efficacy and safety of any agent in MS.

Steps in MS Clinical Trials

Scientific Rationale

Both scientific rigor and the rules of regulatory agencies such as the Food and Drug Administration, and related agencies in Canada and Europe dictate a set path for development and testing new treatments for human diseases. These include demonstration of biologic relevance, safety, and efficacy in a stepwise fashion that can take many years to accomplish.

There must be a strong scientific rationale for being tested in this disease. Based on our knowledge of the MS process and on prior experimental studies of the drug in the laboratory, in animal disease models for MS, or in human disorders with similarities to MS, scientists will conclude that a drug may have a potential role in the treatment or management of MS. The drug likely will have no impact on disease outcome and will be wasteful of the time and effort of participating individuals with MS and their physicians, as well as the financial resources required for the study. Many "alternative" therapies can be faulted on this first criterion: a lack of bona fide biologic rationale for even being considered in a disease such as MS.

If a scientific rationale has developed for a potential therapy, it goes through a detailed set of "preclinical" studies, either in laboratory Petri dishes and test tubes (in vitro) or in living animals (in vivo) to better understand the action of the agent, the pharmacologic dynamics of its use, and its safety in a setting in which humans are not yet exposed to the agent. Such preclinical testing usually continues even after an agent has been given to humans for evaluation.

"Preliminary" or Phase 1 Studies

Given a strong scientific rationale and acceptable results from preclinical testing in laboratory and animal research, human trials almost always begin with toxicity or safety studies in a very small number of people with the disease. This is a "preliminary" or *phase 1* clinical trial. In such early experiments, physicians look for evidence that the agent is safe for use in humans—the most vital consideration in any medical intervention. If such studies demonstrate that the agent is safe, a physician may pursue further studies to get a sense of possible efficacy. Phase 1 studies will also often begin to explore different doses or routes of delivery (e.g., oral, injection) of the experimental agent, to help define the safety and tolerability spectrum of the agent.

"Pilot" or Phase 2 Clinical Trials

These studies usually involve larger, statistically relevant numbers of patients (often twenty to 250 or more) to assess key factors such as:

1. Determining the effectiveness of the drug in halting progression, reducing relapse rate, or improving symptoms and function;
2. Obtaining additional information about toxicity and safety; and
3. Refining knowledge about the best possible dose and route of delivery.

Such pilot studies aim to be objective in obtaining the required answers. We need to compare patient performance while on these drugs with a person's pre-drug status or against the known performance of a similar group of individuals not receiving treatment. Even better, patients on the trial drug might be compared with an identical group of patients who are on a parallel "control" track but being given sham or placebo treatment when ethically and practically possible, or with patients who are being actively treated with the existing best available therapy for that form of disease.

True objectivity is enhanced in controlled studies if both the patients and the physicians are "blinded" or "masked" to the treatment status of individual subjects. In other words, neither knows which group of patients is receiving the experimental drug and which group is being given control treatment. Such "double-blinded" studies are hard to achieve, given the fact that many test agents have side effects that may be "unblinding" to the patient or examining physician. Also, some therapies are hard to hide if the patient gets injections on one schedule compared to a treatment that is oral or by a different injection route or schedule. But rigorous efforts at blinding are essential to reduce the likelihood of bias.

Increasingly, phase 1 and 2 studies are being combined into a "phase 1-2" study to speed the initial assessment of toxicity and efficacy. Magnetic resonance imaging (MRI) to detect the impact of treatment on lesion development in the central nervous system is now used as a key outcome in such studies in MS, and often is the primary outcome that is monitored. MRI is an effective marker of disease activity and disease pathology, and since MRI changes tend to occur relatively rapidly compared with more difficult-to-detect clinical changes they can shorten a trial if MRI change is taken as the outcome. If another outcome, such as reduction of disability, is measured, the studies are longer and MRI would be used for assessment of secondary outcomes.

Results from such phase 1-2 studies can often take several years to obtain. They may or may not show statistical benefit to people receiving the drug compared with people receiving control therapy, and may or may not show acceptable levels of side effects and tolerability. An experimental agent usually is abandoned as a possible therapy if there is no benefit, or if there are uncontrollable or dangerous side effects. On the other hand, if the possibility of benefit remains after the study, and side effects are acceptable, a further clinical trial, usually with a primary focus on change in clinical status, will be undertaken to confirm and expand the studies.

"Definitive" or Phase 3 Clinical Trials

These trials usually are the final step toward making a decision about the value of a proposed therapy. As in phase 2 studies, the key questions are efficacy and safety. Large, statistically determined numbers of participants are essential, and the study often is conducted at a number of different sites and often is international in scope to ensure that the drug can be used in an equivalent fashion by many physicians in many care settings. These studies require large numbers of patients over a long period and are very expensive.

Rigorous adherence to blinding of patients and examining physicians is essential. Randomization of patients to the study and the control group is essential so that the groups are as similar in all meaningful ways as possible. Investigators try to pick patients similar in age, sex distribution, type, duration and degree of disability. At the conclusion of the study period, when the blinding code is broken and the performance of drug-treated patients can be compared with that of the control group patients, there should be sufficient information to determine if the tested agent is truly safe and effective. Phase 3 studies in MS virtually always track the impact of an experimental agent on measurable change in the patient and additional studies might be added as "secondary outcomes" of interest. In order to achieve regulatory acceptance, it is required that the therapy has an impact on the clinical course of the disease.

Recent definitive clinical trials for MS have included as many as 1,500 individuals or more, have involved fifty to one hundred or more participating centers, often distributed around the world, and have taken multiple years to complete. These are the "gold standard" studies from which physicians and patients may have the best confidence that the results are sound.

There are variations in these study designs, often depending on the amount of information available about a new drug from the laboratory, from use in other diseases, or from prior use in MS. Not all new agents go through a test phase in animal models of MS. And in some cases, phase 2 and phase 3 studies are combined into a single large phase 2-3 study when there is sufficient information available from previous studies on dosing and route of delivery. These are also the elements and data required by the Food and Drug Administration and similar regulatory bodies in many countries, which closely monitor clinical trials at every step. It is ultimately the regulatory authority's assessment of the results of benefit and safety and the care with which a study is done that determines whether any agent may be marketed as a treatment for MS.

"Postmarketing" or Phase 4 Studies

Once governmental regulatory approval has been granted and a new agent can be marketed and advertised as a treatment for MS, there often is a series of further studies, which are termed "post-marketing" or *phase 4* studies. These usually are designed to collect long-term information about safety and adverse reactions to the agent, to evaluate its continued efficacy over time, and to explore the use of the drug for different forms of disease.

In some cases, regulatory authorities mandate phase 4 studies to collect data that were missing or insufficient in the definitive analysis and that are important in understanding the use of the new medication. Sometimes the outcome of these mandated phase 4 studies can determine continued marketability of new agents. Should data become available that change the original understanding of the safety and efficacy of the new agent and compromise its use, regulatory authorities may remove the treatment from the market.

Financing Clinical Trials

Drug studies are time consuming and expensive. Such studies most often are supported financially by pharmaceutical and biotechnology companies that invest significant "research and development" resources in these experiments. Grants from the federal government or voluntary health agencies, such as the National Multiple Sclerosis Society and its counterparts around the world, also may fund part or all of the cost of clinical trials. It is rare (and often considered unethical) to request that a patient who volunteers to participate as an experimental subject be asked to pay for that privilege.

Who Participates in Clinical Trials?

The decision for any person with MS to participate in an experimental clinical trial is an intensely personal one and is highly subjective. Since there is always the potential for risk of any untested agent, a potential study participant must be fully informed by the treating physician with a clear assessment of the potential risk factors in the study. Informed consent, including close personal discussion with the physician and nurse as well as required written permission from the study participant, is a legal requirement that protects the rights of all participants.

A true sense of altruism, coupled with a sense of adventure, often characterize those who volunteer to participate in such studies, since participation in either an active treatment or sham group ultimately may help tens of thousands of people with MS. The clinical trial volunteer is a true hero.

Why Can't Some Patients Participate in Clinical Trials?

Disappointed patients will ask, "Doctor, why can't I be in your clinical trial?"

Clinical trials generally are limited to a fixed number of individuals, who must be located geographically close to one of the clinical centers where the study is undertaken. Since most studies require intense and frequent clinic visits at specific predetermined times throughout several years, difficulties in travel from home to the clinic may be considered in determining whether someone will be accepted into a study.

The design of trials is such that generally only one type of MS—for instance, relapsing-remitting disease—is involved in the study. This excludes people with any other form of MS. Even within the group of interest, further restrictions, called inclusion and exclusion criteria, will be enforced in virtually all studies: disease limited to a certain duration or a certain level of disability; restricted age of participants; exclusions based on prior medications or participation in previous trials of agents for which there might be dangerous or confusing effects with the new experimental treatment.

For any particular test drug, other restrictions also may apply, depending on the known characteristics of the test medication. There are often prohibitions against pregnancy as new drugs don't yet have safety information about the mother or fetus. Some medical conditions cause confusion with MS symptoms or add medications that would confuse the record of side effects from the new drug. If a patient is disappointed by not being entered in a trial, they may take some solace from the realization that positive findings eventually are available to all patients

Where Can I Learn About Ongoing Clinical Trials?

Finding out about clinical trials in MS should be a joint project of the patient and the physician. The network of physicians who organize and participate in MS clinical trials is ever growing, and in consultation with a personal physician, an interested patient usually can learn of any pending studies locally or in nearby communities, often with the assistance of the local branch or chapter of the National Multiple Sclerosis Society, Multiple Sclerosis Society of Canada, or their over thirty affiliated member organizations around the world. The U.S. National Multiple Sclerosis Society (www.nationalmssociety.org) has an extensive listing of ongoing and newly recruiting MS clinical trials in the United States and elsewhere, as does the Consortium of Multiple Sclerosis Centers (www.mscare.org) through its NARCOMS affiliate group; the Multiple Sclerosis International Federation (www.msif.org) carries similar information about trials around the world. Other sources, which might include information about MS clinical trials but are not specific or restricted to MS, include Centerwatch (www .centerwatch.com) and the U.S. Department of Health and Human Services (www.clincaltrials.gov).

CHAPTER 12

How Multiple Sclerosis Organizations Can Help

People with MS have many needs and concerns related to their diagnosis and struggles with MS, and some of these are shared by family members and close friends. The issues are different at different stages of the disease, the nature of the symptoms or disability, and the family and work situation. The needs will also vary due to the different personality characteristics, previous life events, and learning and coping styles of the individuals.

The family physician or neurologist is a frequent source of information. While this is certainly appropriate for issues related to the disease symptoms and treatment, a medical practice is not an adequate resource to accommodate the extensive nonmedical needs of those with MS, their families, friends, and other concerned persons such as employers, teachers, and health professionals. In North America, the primary resources for addressing nonmedical MS-related needs are the National Multiple Sclerosis Society in the United States and the Multiple Sclerosis Society of Canada, the

Multiple Sclerosis Association of America, the Multiple Sclerosis Foundation, the Consortium of Multiple Sclerosis Centers, the International Organization of Multiple Sclerosis Nurses, Can Do MS, and the Multiple Sclerosis Coalition. This chapter provides general information about these organizations, as well as the specific ways these organizations can help you.

The National Multiple Sclerosis Society

The National Multiple Sclerosis Society (NMSS) was the first non-profit organization in the United States to support national and international research on the prevention, cure, and treatment of MS. Equally important, the Society's goals include the provision of nationwide programs to assist people with MS and their families and the provision of information about MS to those with the disease, family members, professionals, and the public. Programs are designed to help people with MS to maintain their independence and lifestyle. The Society's mission—to end the devastating effects of MS—addresses the negative impact of the disease in the present through education and services to support a positive quality of life and into the future through research and advocacy.

The NMSS was founded in 1946 by Sylvia Lawry, whose brother had MS. In her search to learn more about the disease, she found that very few people in the country professed any interest in the disease. Ms. Lawry placed an advertisement in *The New York Times* seeking any information about successful treatments for MS. A number of people who were also touched by MS responded. They had no news of a cure, but asked that Ms. Lawry share whatever helpful information she received. And so the National Multiple Sclerosis Society was born.

The NMSS continues to grow. A fifty-state network of chapters provides assistance and education. The home offices in New York City, Denver, and Washington, DC, direct MS-related research and advocacy, provide some specific services, and provide support, structure, and guidance for chapters. Policies and national priorities are established by a National Board of Directors, composed of business and professional leaders with a special interest in MS. The Board is assisted by a nationally representative group of individuals with MS, the National Programs Advisory Council. Each local chapter is governed by a Board of Trustees. Staff at both national and chapter levels work in partnership with volunteers and the community to implement the necessary and desired programs. There is an ongoing process of identifying needs and eliciting feedback regarding the value of programs. This involves people with MS, their families, and the professionals who serve them, and provides direction for Society activities.

Philosophy of NMSS Programs

The NMSS and its chapters are committed to empowering people with MS to live as independently as possible within the limits of their disabilities and to the maximum of their capabilities within the least restrictive environment. This goal is achieved through programs, services, and activities that:

- Promote and support knowledge, health, and independence
- Inform and educate people with MS and their families, professionals, public officials, and the general public about MS
- Provide support programs that help people with MS and their families cope with the changes and challenges that MS presents
- Help people gain access to community resources and quality specialty health care
- Stimulate changes and developments in the community and public policy beneficial to people affected by MS
- Fill gaps in community resources

The Society believes that all people with MS and their families in the United States should have access to certain basic programs and ensures this through its chapter certification process.

All people with MS are offered services without discrimination. Access is not affected by a person's race, color, religion, age, disability, sexual orientation, or the individual's relationship with a chapter. Chapters do hold "targeted" programs to meet the needs of specific groups; for example, education programs for those newly diagnosed, young professionals' groups, and the gay/lesbian community.

The confidentiality of members with MS and their family members ("clients") is strictly maintained.

Who Does the NMSS Serve?

The Society's mission reflects a dedication to "end the devastating effects of multiple sclerosis." At the center of chapter programs are people who have MS. Since the disease affects others as well, NMSS clients are all who come to the Society for information and/or professional assistance. The secondary focus of its programs is the MS "family circle"—spouses, children, parents, relatives, and significant others. Coworkers and close friends are included in this circle as well. Family members and significant others can also utilize chapter programs.

The NMSS is a leading source of information on MS for the general public. It also provides education to health professionals, service providers, and community agencies. This information and education can have significant impact on quality of life, increasing access to quality health care and community resources, and promoting understanding from others.

Quality of Life Goals

The NMSS organizes services under three main Quality of Life Goals: MS Knowledge, Health, and Independence. Specific services are addressed within this framework.

Knowledge

The NMSS facilitates the acquisition of essential knowledge about MS by providing information and education to clients, families, professionals, and the public. Information is the first and most frequent request the NMSS receives from people with MS. Client surveys consistently request more information about MS: symptoms, diagnosis, programs, treatment, research, and related issues such as employment, health insurance, disability rights, and family issues.

Seeking information about MS is usually a first step in the coping process. Getting accurate up-to-date information can assist you to make informed decisions, become aware of needs and resources, and take some control over this unpredictable and complex disease. One of the main functions of the NMSS is to serve as the repository of the most current and accurate information on MS. This includes:

- Information can be obtained by calling 1-800-FIGHT-MS (1-800-344-4867)

- Website with updated information about treatments, current research, and programs (http://www.nationalmssociety.org)

- *Knowledge Is Power* educational program (serial mailings) for people newly diagnosed with MS and their families, available through all chapters or on the website

- *Moving Forward* group educational program for people newly diagnosed with MS and their families

- Educational programs on various topics throughout the year

- Annual national education program

- Booklets, articles, and information sheets on MS-related topics (see Resources)

- Lending library of books, audio- and/or videotapes, with mail access

- *Inside* MS national bimonthly magazine plus chapter newsletter issued quarterly or more often

Health

The NMSS helps people with MS to achieve optimal health physically, emotionally, and in their relationships.

PHYSICAL HEALTH

People with MS must deal with concerns about physical impairments related to the disease and their impact on general physical health. NMSS programs and services address physical health needs by:

- Promoting state-of-the-art MS health care and facilitating access for people with MS through formal affiliations with MS clinical facilities and professional education programs
- Providing referrals to neurologists, physical therapists, and other medical/rehabilitation professionals knowledgeable about MS
- Swimming and other exercise programs sponsored or co-sponsored by some chapters or referral to existing programs in the community
- Wellness programs
- Affiliation with local MS clinical facilities to facilitate access to, and coordination of, health services
- Participation in local and national advocacy issues related to physical health, for example, health insurance reform, through Action Alert Network. (Call your local chapter to join or sign up on the Society's website.)

EMOTIONAL HEALTH

Emotional health is a state of psychological well-being, including an individual's adaptive capacities. It is demonstrated by successful interactions with others and with the social environment. Difficulties with adaptation to a chronic illness are normal and respond favorably to a variety of interventions.

Although NMSS chapters are not primarily mental health agencies, they can help individuals and their significant others in their adaptation to chronic illness. Chapters provide short-term counseling: defined as "reflective listening and problem solving." The social isolation that often results from having a chronic illness can be reduced through peer relationships and group programs that bring people together.

NMSS chapters offer assistance with problem solving, including:

- *"Someone to Listen"* peer support program, which meets the second most requested service—to speak with another person who has MS. "Peers" are specially trained to provide information and support to the person with MS.

- Local counselor/therapist referrals.

- Self-help groups—leaders have often received group leadership training through the Society.

- Peer support programs.

FAMILY SUPPORT

Families of people with MS are important to the NMSS, which has formally adopted the Family Service America, Inc. definition of family: "A family consists of two or more people, whether living together or apart, related by blood, marriage, adoption, or commitment to care for one another."

This definition highlights the inclusion of all varieties of family configurations. The NMSS recognizes the enormous, ongoing stress that the entire family experiences, as well as the critical support provided by the family to the person with MS. Programs emphasize the strengths of the family and bolster these strengths by offering education and other means of support and assistance.

The NMSS sponsors a variety of family programs that combine education, counseling, and social activities. Some chapters have family counseling programs, referrals to experienced community counselors in others. The *Children with MS* program provides support, networking, education, and counseling for children/ teens with MS and their parents (call the Denver home office: 303-813-6623).

Independence

The NMSS is committed to promoting the highest possible level of independence for people with MS.

INDEPENDENT LIVING AND ACCESSIBILITY

The NMSS can provide referrals to centers for independent living, equipment vendors, accessible housing, and others.

All chapter offices and program locations are accessible to people with disabilities.

EMPLOYMENT

Referrals and consultations are available to help people continue employment despite MS-related obstacles.

LONG-TERM CARE SERVICES

Programs are available to help people who are moderately to severely limited by MS-related disability receive necessary personal services and other assistance.

The Multiple Sclerosis Society of Canada

Founded in 1948, the Multiple Sclerosis Society of Canada has a growing membership with seven regional divisions and more than 120 chapters. The head office is located in Toronto, Ontario, and division offices are located in Halifax, Montreal, Toronto, Winnipeg, Regina, Edmonton, and Vancouver. The mission is "to be a leader in finding a cure for MS and enabling people affected by MS to enhance their quality of life." The Multiple Sclerosis Society of Canada funds a research program totaling about $6 million annually. It also has a $20 million endMS program to encourage young trainees to have their careers dedicated to MS research.

Client Services

The Multiple Sclerosis Society of Canada provides a wide variety of programs and services for those affected by MS. These include the following.

INFORMATION AND REFERRAL

- Multiple Sclerosis Society of Canada publications
- ASK MS and National Information Resource Centre

- Lending libraries
- Information and referrals over the phone or by email

EDUCATION

- Conferences and workshops

SUPPORT

- Individual advocacy
- Support and self-help groups
- Recreation and social programs

ADVOCACY

- Helping individuals with MS obtain needed services

FUNDING

- Equipment purchase or loan programs
- Special assistance programs

Services vary across the country depending on the kind of provincial government and community programs available, since the Society does not duplicate services available through other sources. The Society currently spends nearly $9 million annually on services and education programs for people who have MS, their family members, and all others affected by MS.

Awareness Activities

The Multiple Sclerosis Society of Canada is firmly committed to informing Canadians about MS and how they can join the fight against MS. The national office coordinates an overall public awareness campaign that is complemented by division and chapter activities.

Government Relations/Social Action

The Multiple Sclerosis Society of Canada works with people who have MS to ensure that they have the opportunity to participate fully in all aspects of life. Volunteers across the country endeavor to change government policies at all levels, private industry practices, and public attitudes in ways that will positively benefit people with MS.

Fund Raising

The Multiple Sclerosis Society of Canada has growing total revenues annually. The funds are used to support research, client services, public education, social action, and volunteer resources. Most of this income comes from public donations, bequests, and special fund-raising programs conducted by the Society. The major fund-raising programs are the MS Carnation Campaign, the RONA MS Bike Tour, the MS Read-A-Thon, the Super Cities WALK for MS, the direct marketing program, and major gifts/planned giving.

History

A small group of dedicated volunteers in Montreal founded the Multiple Sclerosis Society of Canada in 1948 after contact with the newly established National Multiple Sclerosis Society in the United States. Support of MS research began in 1949.

Headquarters for the Society remained in Montreal until the mid-1960s, when the offices were moved to Toronto. Other advances came with the establishment of regional divisions; there are now seven divisions across Canada from coast to coast. The Multiple Sclerosis International Federation, of which the Canadian Society is a charter member, was established in 1967.

MS Clinics

The Multiple Sclerosis Society of Canada is proud to work with a network of specialized MS clinics across the country. Clinic services vary, but most offer a wide range of services, delivered by a multidisciplinary health care team. These services usually include:

- Expert diagnostic and treatment services for people with MS

- Clinical research, especially in the area of MS treatment options

- Educational and support programs for people with MS and their families and caregivers

To learn more about the clinic in your area and the services it provides, contact the Multiple Sclerosis Society of Canada for contact information on the clinic in your area by calling toll-free in Canada at 1-800-268-7582.

The Multiple Sclerosis Association of America

The Multiple Sclerosis Association of America (MSAA) is a national nonprofit organization founded in 1970 dedicated to enriching the quality of life for everyone affected by MS. The MSAA provides ongoing support and direct services to individuals with MS and people close to them. It also serves to promote greater understanding of the needs and challenges of those who face physical obstacles. Its philosophy and effort have focused on enriching the quality of day-to-day living for everyone affected by MS. It helps each individual on a personal level and relies on volunteers and support from the general public. The MSAA's national office in Cherry Hill, New Jersey, serves clients throughout the United States. Its regional offices, the Midwest Regional Office, Northwest Regional Office, Southeast Regional Office, Northeast Regional Office, South—Central Regional Office and Western Regional Office, provide additional assistance on a more local basis, facilitating outreach and awareness. Regional offices conduct awareness and educational conferences and workshops and bring people together through networking and events and conduct fundraising activities. Overseeing MSAA's activities is a national Board of Directors comprised of accomplished professionals from across the country, volunteering their time. Providing medical consultation is MSAA's Chief Medical Officer, who reviews all of MSAA's medical information and chairs its Healthcare Advisory Council, which brings significant leadership, knowledge, and expertise in the fields of neurology, nursing, and physical therapy and provides strategic support and guidance on health-related issues.

Vital Programs and Services

MSAA's website (http://www.msassociation.org) is an excellent resource for anyone interested in learning more about MS featuring topics such as "What is MS," "Types of MS," and "Treatments of MS." There is a "Newly Diagnosed" section offering answers and support. MSAA publications provide a great deal of helpful and important information and cover a wide range of subjects such as medical research and treatments, symptom management, complementary and alternative therapies, as well as general information. Its national magazine, *The Motivator*, includes articles on vital issues such as new research, treatments, and personal stories. All publications are available free of charge and may be viewed, downloaded, or ordered at www.msassociation.org or by calling toll-free 1-800-532-7667. The Lending Library offers a collection of nearly 300 MS resources on diagnosis, symptoms, treatments, general health, along with books that inspire through personal experiences and life stories. MSAA loans and mails the books and DVDs free of charge, along with instructions for returning them free of charge.

MSAA provides people with MS with equipment ranging from grab bars to wheelchairs; cooling accessories for heat-sensitive individuals; a mobile phone app, *My MS Manager*, for use free of charge on an iPhone, iPad or iPod touch. Visit http://www.msassociation .org/mobile to download *My MS Manager*. A new program called S.E.A.R.C.H has been introduced to assist the MS community about different treatment choices. It is designed as a memory aid, the acronym representing the key areas that need to be discussed with one's health care team when "searching" for the most appropriate MS treatment. S.E.A.R.C.H. stands for safety, effectiveness, affordability, risks, convenience, and health outcomes. Written materials about the program can be downloaded at http://www.msassociation.org/search or requested at 1-800-532-7667.

MSAA provides assistance in acquiring magnetic resonance imaging (MRI) scans for patients without insurance or who have been denied coverage for an MRI. The *Staying Connected* program is a networking program that facilitates peer support. It is an online community of individuals with MS and their care partners who are interested in corresponding via email with others who are affected by MS. Email correspondence through this program is especially helpful for those who are unable to attend traditional support group meetings but want to stay connected to the MS community. The *Staying Connected* network program's online directory is password protected and available through MSAA's website.

The Multiple Sclerosis Foundation

The Multiple Sclerosis Foundation (MSF) provides a comprehensive approach to helping people with MS maintain their health and well-being by offering programming and support to keep them self-sufficient and their homes safe, and by conduction educational programs to heighten public awareness and promote understanding about the disease. MSF is a service-based, non-profit organization with national headquarters in Fort Lauderdale, Florida. It serves the nation from one central location eliminating the need for branch offices in order to maintain a more cost-effective and efficient operation while maintaining the highest quality service. It networks with independent, grassroots organizations to give it a local presence in communities around the nation.

The MSF was established in 1986. It is a publicly funded 501 organization and the funds it raises go directly into services designed to improve the quality of life for people with MS. All of its services including information, literature, and subscriptions to its publications are provided free of charge. Some programs are needs-based and dependent on income and other factors while other programs are available to all individuals affected by MS. The MSF sponsors Home Care Grant Programs, Support Groups, Peer Counseling, and a yearly Cruise for the Cause where people with MS and their families cruise together to interact with MS health care professionals to gain knowledge about MS and support. It has a Lending Library and excellent publications on the different aspects of MS for patients and their families. Information about MSF programs can be obtained by calling 1-888-MSFOCUS or on its website, http://www.msfocus.org.

The Consortium of MS Centers

The Consortium of MS Centers (CMSC) is an organization of MS health care providers intent on improving the lives of those affected by MS. Its members are neurologists, nurses, physical therapists, neuropsychologists, and social workers who work with MS patients. It was organized in 1986 under the direction of neurologists interested in the clinical care of MS. It has grown to become a multidisciplinary organization providing a team approach to MS care and a network for all health care professionals and others specializing in the care of persons with MS. It has over 200 member centers in the United States, Canada, and Europe, representing over 4,000 health care professionals worldwide who provide care for more than 150,000 individuals with MS.

CMSC provides leadership in clinical research and education; develops vehicles to share information and knowledge among members; disseminates information to the health care community and to persons affected by MS.. Through its CMSC North American Research Committee on Multiple Sclerosis (NARCOMS) based at the University of Alabama at Birmingham, it maintains a patient registry, website, expert forum and research registry to promote MS research. It has an online journal, the *International Journal of Multiple Sclerosis Care*, to promote multi-disciplinary approaches to treating persons with MS. While this is an organization for health care professionals rather than patients, patients will find articles of interest to them on its website (http://www.mscare.org).

The International Organization of Multiple Sclerosis Nurses

The International Organization of Multiple Sclerosis Nurses (IOMSN) was founded on May 30, 1997 and is the first and only international organization focusing solely on the needs and goals of professional nurses, anywhere in the world, who care for people with MS. By mentoring, educating, networking, sharing—the IOMSN supports nurses in their continuing effort to offer hope. The IOMSN establishes standards of nursing care in MS, supports research, and educates the health care community about MS.

Out of this group came the development of an examination to certify nurses who provide MS care. This is a group that those of you with MS will want your nurses to join. While it is only for MS nurses, its website will provide information helpful to patients and connect you to other sites that will be of interest. The website is http://www.iomsn.org.

Can Do MS

Can Do MS is a leading provider of innovative lifestyle empow- erment programs for people with MS and their support partners. Leveraging the powerful legacy and principles of former Olympian and organizational founder, Jimmie Heuga, Can Do MS has helped thousands of people living with MS reclaim a sense of dignity, con- trol, and freedom by empowering them with the knowledge, skills, tools and confidence to transform challenges into possibilities.

Can Do MS does programs all over the United States but it also has events and webinars listed on their website at http://www .mscando.org.

The MS Coalition

The MS Coalition (MSC) is another organization that benefits peo- ple who have MS. It was founded in 2005 by three independent MS organizations, the MSAA, the MSF and the NMSS, in an effort to work together to benefit individuals with MS. Since that time it has grown to a nine-member organization, all of whom provide critical MS programs and services. Its members are the Multiple Sclerosis Association of America (MSAA), the Multiple Sclerosis

Foundation (MSF), the National Multiple Sclerosis Society (NMSS), the United Spinal Association, Accelerated Cure Project for Multiple Sclerosis, The Consortium of Multiple Sclerosis Centers (CMSC), Can Do MS, and the International Organization of Multiple Sclerosis Nurses (IOMSN). It is important for you to know about this organization because its vision is to improve the quality of life for those affected by MS through a collaborative network of independent MS organizations. Its mission is to increase opportunities for cooperation and provide greater opportunity to leverage the effective use of resources for the benefit of the MS community.

The first chapter of this book began by making you aware of the history of MS. Hopefully you will realize from its other chapters how far we have come. In the coming years you will note that we continue to have rapid improvements in the treatment of the disease as we move forward to work for better treatments and a cure.

Glossary

ACTIVITIES OF DAILY LIVING (ADLs)
ADLs include any daily activity a person performs for self-care (feeding, grooming, bathing, dressing), work, homemaking, and leisure. The ability to perform ADLs is often used as a measure of ability/ disability in MS.

ACUTE
Having a rapid or sudden onset.

ACUTE DISSEMINATED ENCEPHALOMYELITIS (ADEM)
A demyelinating disorder, usually in children, usually following a viral infection and rarely vaccination. The clinical features and MRI may resemble MS, but the disorder usually happens in one acute event. Oligoclonal bans are usually absent in the cerebral spinal fluid, which is helpful in separating this from MS, and if there are bans, they are only in the acute phase and then disappear, whereas they persist in MS.

ADRENOCORTICOTROPIC HORMONE (ACTH)

A naturally occurring pituitary hormone that stimulates the adrenal gland to produce corticosteroids. It was uses to treat acute attacks of MS in the past but has mostly been replaced by methylprednisolone, and is not easily available now.

ANTIBODIES (Ab)

Immunoglobulins or large Y-shaped proteins of the immune system that are primarily produced by plasma cells and used by the immune system to identify and neutralize pathogens such as viruses and bacteria, and also proteins recognized as "foreign" antigens. *See* Antigen.

ANTICHOLINERGIC

Refers to the action of certain medications commonly used in the management of neurogenic bladder dysfunction. These medications inhibit the transmission of parasympathetic nerve impulses and thereby reduce spasms of smooth muscle in the bladder.

ANTIGEN

Any substance that triggers the immune system to produce an antibody; generally refers to infectious organisms, toxic substances, or proteins the immune system identifies as being "foreign". *See* Antibodies.

ASSISTIVE DEVICES

Any tools that are designed, fabricated, and/or adapted to assist a person in performing a particular task (e.g., cane, walker, shower chair, adapted kitchen utensils).

ATAXIA

The incoordination and unsteadiness that result from the brain's failure to regulate the body's posture and the strength and direction of limb movements. Ataxia is most often caused by disease activity in the cerebellum.

AUTOIMMUNE DISEASE

An immune system malfunction in which the body's immune system causes illness by attacking its own cells, organs, or tissues. Multiple sclerosis is believed to be an autoimmune disease, along with systemic lupus erythematosus, rheumatoid arthritis, scleroderma, and many others.

AUTONOMIC NERVOUS SYSTEM

The part of the nervous system that regulates "involuntary" vital functions, including the activity of the cardiac (heart) muscle, blood vessels, smooth muscles (e.g., of the bladder and bowel), and glands.

AXON

The extension of a nerve cell that conducts impulses to other nerve cells or muscles.

B CELL

A type of lymphocyte (white blood cell) manufactured in the bone marrow that makes antibodies.

BABINSKI REFLEX

A neurologic sign in MS in which stroking the outside sole of the foot with a pointed object causes an upward (extensor) movement of the big toe rather than the normal (flexor) downward movement of the toes. It indicates an abnormality in the motor tracks of the central nervous system. *See* Sign.

BLOOD-BRAIN BARRIER

A semipermeable cell layer around blood vessels in the brain and spinal cord that prevents large molecules, immune cells, and potentially damaging substances and disease-causing organisms (e.g., viruses) from passing out of the bloodstream into the central nervous system (brain and spinal cord). A break in the blood-brain barrier may underlie the disease process in MS by allowing immune cells to enter.

BRAIN ATROPHY

Shrinkage of the brain that seems to be due, at least in part, to the loss of myelin and axons. Evidence of atrophy is present in most patients when they have their initial symptoms of MS, indicating the disease has been going on long before. It continues during the disease but therapies can slow this process.

BRAINSTEM

The part of the central nervous system that houses the nerve centers of the head as well as the centers for respiration and heart control. It is the area between the base of the brain and the spinal cord.

CATHETER, URINARY

A hollow, flexible tube, made of plastic or rubber, which can be inserted through the urinary opening into the bladder to drain urine.

CENTRAL NERVOUS SYSTEM

The part of the nervous system that includes the brain, brainstem, spinal cord, and optic nerves.

CEREBELLUM

A part of the brain situated in the brain stem that controls balance and coordination of movement.

CEREBROSPINAL FLUID (CSF)

A watery, colorless, clear fluid that bathes and protects the brain and spinal cord. The composition of this fluid can be altered by a variety of diseases. Certain changes in the CSF that are characteristic of MS can be detected with a lumbar puncture (spinal tap), a test sometimes used to help make the MS diagnosis.

CEREBRUM

The large, upper part of the brain, with two halves (hemispheres) responsible for thought, memory, sensation, and motor movements.

CLINICAL FINDING

An observation made during a medical examination indicating change or impairment in a physical or mental function.

CLINICALLY ISOLATED SYNDROME (CIS)

A first neurological event (e.g., an episode of optic neuritis) that suggests demyelination in the central nervous system, and is accompanied by several "silent" or asymptomatic lesions on MRI that are typical of MS. Individuals with CIS are at high risk for developing clinically definite MS.

CLONUS

A sign of spasticity in which a repetitive reflex jerking happens in the lower leg when the foot is forcibly pushed from under the forefoot. The stretching evokes a repetitive reflex indicating there is spasticity in the lower leg muscles.

COGNITION

High-level functions carried out by the human brain, including comprehension and formation of speech, visual perception and construction, calculation ability, attention (information processing), memory, and executive functions such as planning, problem-solving, and self-monitoring.

COGNITIVE IMPAIRMENT

Changes in cognitive function caused by trauma or disease process. Some degree of cognitive impairment occurs in approximately 50 to 60 percent of people with MS, with some memory, information processing, and executive functions being the most commonly affected functions.

COGNITIVE REHABILITATION

Techniques designed to improve the functioning of individuals whose cognition is impaired because of physical trauma or disease. Rehabilitation strategies are designed to improve the impaired function via repetitive drills or practice, or to compensate impaired functions that are not likely to improve. Cognitive rehabilitation is provided by psychologists and neuropsychologists, speech/language therapists, and occupational therapists. While these three types of specialists use different assessment tools and treatment strategies, they share the common goal of attempting to improve the individual's ability to function as independently and safely as possible in the home and work environment.

COMPUTED TOMOGRAPHY (CT SCAN)

A noninvasive diagnostic radiology technique. A computer integrates x-ray scanned "slices" of the organ being examined into a cross-sectional picture.

CONTRACTION, MUSCLE

A shortening of muscle fibers and muscle that produces movement around a joint.

COORDINATION

An organized working together of muscles and groups of muscles aimed at bringing about an accurate and coordinated purposeful movement such as walking or standing or reaching for an object.

CORTICOSTEROIDS

See Glucocorticoid hormones.

CORTISONE

A glucocorticoid steroid hormone, produced by the adrenal glands or synthetically, that has anti-inflammatory and immune-system suppressing properties. Prednisone, prednisolone, and methylprednisolone also belong to this group of substances used in MS to decrease the duration of attacks.

CRANIAL NERVES

Twelve nerves that carry sensory or motor fibers to the face and neck. Included among this group of twelve nerves are the optic nerves (vision), auditory nerves (hearing), trigeminal nerves (sensation along the face and tongue), olfactory nerves (smell), and vagus nerves (pharynx and vocal cords). Evaluation of cranial nerve function is part of the standard neurological exam.

DEEP TENDON REFLEXES

The involuntary jerks that are normally produced at certain spots on a limb when the tendons are tapped in a way that stretches them, usually with a reflex hammer. Reflexes are tested as part of the standard neurological exam.

DEMYELINATION

A loss of myelin in the white matter of the nervous system.

DIPLOPIA

Double vision, or the simultaneous awareness of two images of the same object that results from a failure of the two eyes to work in a coordinated fashion. Covering one eye will erase one of the images.

DISABILITY

As defined by the World Health Organization, a disability (resulting from an impairment) is a restriction or lack of ability to perform an activity in the manner or within the range considered normal for a human being.

DOUBLE-BLIND CLINICAL STUDY

A study in which none of the participants, including experimental subjects, examining doctors, attending nurses, or any other research staff, know who is taking the test drug and who is taking a control or placebo agent. The purpose of this research design is to avoid bias of the test results. In all studies, safety procedures are designed to "break the blind" if medical circumstances require it.

DYSESTHESIA

Distorted or unpleasant sensations experienced by a person when the skin is touched.

ELECTROENCEPHALOGRAPHY (EEG)

A diagnostic procedure that records, via electrodes attached to various areas of the person's head, electrical activity generated by brain cells. It is particularly important to detect evidence of seizure activity.

ELECTROMYOGRAPHY (EMG)

A diagnostic procedure that records muscle electrical potentials through electrodes. It is often combined with tests of the conduction in the sensory and motor nerves.

ETIOLOGY

The study of all factors that may be involved in the cause of a disease, including the patient's susceptibility, the nature of the disease-causing agent, and the way in which the person's body is invaded by the agent.

EVOKED POTENTIALS (EPs)

Recordings of the nervous system's electrical response to the stimulation of specific sensory pathways (e.g., visual, auditory, general sensory). EPs can demonstrate lesions along specific nerve pathways whether or not the lesions are producing symptoms, thus making this test useful in confirming the diagnosis of MS.

EXACERBATION

The appearance of new symptoms or the aggravation of old ones (synonymous with attack, relapse, flare-up, or worsening); usually associated with inflammation and demyelination in the brain or spinal cord.

EXPERIMENTAL ALLERGIC ENCEPHALOMYELITIS (EAE)

An autoimmune disease resembling MS that is induced in genetically susceptible research animals. Before testing on humans, a potential treatment for MS may first be tested on laboratory animals with EAE in order to suggest the treatment's efficacy and safety in humans. EAE is not MS but resembles it enough to be used as a model for many aspects of MS.

EXTENSOR SPASM

A symptom of spasticity in which the legs straighten suddenly into a stiff, extended position. These spasms, which typically last for several minutes, occur most commonly in bed at night or on rising from bed.

FLACCID

A decrease in muscle tone resulting in loose, "floppy" limbs.

FLEXOR SPASM

Involuntary, sometimes painful contractions of the flexor muscles, which pull the legs upward into a clenched position. They often occur during sleep, but can also occur when the person is in a seated position.

FOOD AND DRUG ADMINISTRATION (FDA)

The U.S. federal agency that is responsible for establishing and enforcing governmental regulations pertaining to the manufacture and sale of food, drugs, and cosmetics. Its role is to certify benefits of medication and prevent the sale of impure or dangerous substances. Any new drug that is proposed for the treatment of MS must be approved by the FDA.

FOOT DROP

A condition of weakness in the muscles of the foot and ankle, caused by poor nerve conduction, which interferes with a person's ability to elevate the forefoot, producing a dragging of the foot when walking. The toes touch the ground before the heel, and may cause the person to trip or lose balance.

FRONTAL LOBES

The anterior (front) part of each of the cerebral hemispheres that make up the cerebrum. The back part of the frontal lobe is the motor cortex, which controls voluntary movement; the area of the frontal lobe that is further forward is concerned with learning, behavior, judgment, and personality.

GLUCOCORTICOID HORMONES

Steroid hormones that are produced by the adrenal glands in response to stimulation by adrenocorticotropic hormone (ACTH) from the pituitary. These hormones, which can also be manufactured synthetically (prednisone, prednisolone, methylprednisolone, betamethasone, dexamethasone), serve both an immunosuppressive and an anti-inflammatory role in the treatment of MS exacerbations: They help control overactive immune response and interfere with the release of certain inflammation-producing enzymes.

HANDICAP

As defined by the World Health Organization, a handicap is a disadvantage, resulting from an impairment and disability, that interferes with a person's efforts to fulfill a role that is normal for that person. Handicap is therefore a social concept, representing the social and environmental consequences of a person's impairments and disabilities.

HELPER T-LYMPHOCYTES

White blood cells that are a major contributor to the immune system's inflammatory response against myelin.

IMMUNE SYSTEM

A complex system of cells and dissolvable proteins that protect the body against disease-producing organisms and other foreign invaders.

IMMUNOCOMPETENT CELLS
White blood cells (B and T lymphocytes and others) that defend against invading agents in the body.

IMMUNOSUPPRESSION
In MS, a form of treatment that slows or inhibits the body's natural immune responses, including those directed against the body's own tissues. Examples of immunosuppressive treatments in MS include cyclophosphamide, cyclosporine, methotrexate, and azathioprine.

IMPAIRMENT
As defined by the World Health Organization, an impairment is any loss of function directly resulting from injury or disease.

INCIDENCE
The number of new cases of a disease in a specified population over a defined period of time. It is often used in a form of the number of cases in a defined population (such as 100,000) in a year.

INCONTINENCE
The inability to control passage of urine or feces.

INFLAMMATION
A tissue's immunologic response to injury, characterized by mobilization of white blood cells and antibodies, swelling, and fluid accumulation.

INTENTION TREMOR
Rhythmic shaking that occurs in the course of a purposeful movement, such as reaching to pick something up or bringing an outstretched finger in to touch one's nose.

INTERFERON
A group of immune system proteins, produced and released in the presence of a virus, bacteria, parasite or tumor cells. They modify the body's immune response by activating nearby cells to inhibit the multiplication of viruses. The tendency to interfere with viruses gave rise to the name. The benefits of interferons in therapy relates to its

immune effects, not just to the anti-viral effects. Several interferons have been approved by the Food and Drug Administration for treatment of relapsing-remitting MS.

LUMBAR PUNCTURE

A diagnostic procedure to sample cerebrospinal fluid (CSF) by inserting a hollow needle into the spinal canal in the lumbar area of the lower back. It is often called a spinal tap. The CSF can be tested for various features such as cells, sugar, proteins infectious agents, and in MS, for oligoclonal banding patterns of proteins.

LYMPHOCYTE

A subtype of white blood cells that is part of the immune system. Lymphocytes can be subdivided into B lymphocytes, which originate in the bone marrow and produce antibodies; T lymphocytes, which are produced in the bone marrow and mature in the thymus; and natural killer cells, which can bind to certain tumor and virus infected cells and kill them by inserting granules containing a substance called perforin. Helper T lymphocytes heighten immune responses; suppressor T lymphocytes suppress them.

MACROPHAGE

A white blood cell with scavenger characteristics that ingests and destroys foreign substances, such as bacteria and cell debris.

MAGNETIC RESONANCE IMAGING (MRI)

A diagnostic procedure that produces computer-generated visual images of body parts by using strong magnetic fields. An important diagnostic tool in MS, MRI makes it possible to visualize and count lesions in the white matter of the brain and spinal cord.

MINIMAL RECORD OF DISABILITY (MRD)

A standardized method for quantifying the clinical status of a person with MS. The MRD is made up of five parts: demographic information; the Neurological Functional Systems, which assign scores to clinical findings for each of the various neurological systems in the brain and spinal cord (pyramidal, cerebellar, brainstem, sensory, visual, mental, bowel and bladder); the Disability Status Scale, which gives a single composite score for the person's disease; the Incapacity Status Scale, which is an inventory of functional disabilities relating to activities of daily living; the Environmental Status Scale, which provides an assessment of social handicap resulting from chronic illness. The MRD assist doctors and other professionals in assessing the impact of MS and in planning and coordinating the care of people with MS.

MONOCLONAL ANTIBODIES
Laboratory-produced antibodies, which can be designed to react against a specific antigen in order to alter the immune response.

MOTOR NEURONS
Nerve cells of the brain and spinal cord that enable movement of muscles in various parts of the body.

MUSCLE TONE
A characteristic of a muscle tension brought about by the constant flow of nerve stimuli to that muscle. Abnormal muscle tone can be defined as: hypertonus (increased muscle tone, as in spasticity); hypotonus (reduced muscle tone or flaccid paralysis); or atony (loss of muscle tone). Muscle tone is evaluated as part of the standard neurological exam in MS.

MYELIN
A fatty white coating of nerve fibers in the central nervous system, composed of lipids (fats) and protein. Myelin serves as insulation and as an aid to rapid nerve fiber conduction. When myelin is damaged in MS, nerve fiber conduction is faulty or absent.

MYELIN BASIC PROTEIN
A protein comprising about 30 percent of all myelin of the central nervous system that may be found in higher than normal concentrations in the cerebrospinal fluid of individuals with MS and other diseases that damage myelin. Some believe myelin basic protein is an antigen against which autoimmune responses are triggered in MS.

MYELITIS

An inflammatory disease of the spinal cord. In transverse myelitis, the inflammation spreads across the tissue of the spinal cord, resulting in a loss of its normal function to transmit nerve impulses up and down.

MYELOPATHY

A lesion of the spinal cord that may be partial or complete. It is not uncommon as a presenting feature of MS, and the clinician needs to look for other evidence of lesions elsewhere, clinically, on the MRI and with oligoclonal banding, to confirm MS. (Other terms used are acute or subacute, and transverse myelopathy.)

NERVE

A bundle of nerve fibers (axons). Fibers are either afferent (leading toward the brain and serving in the perception of sensory stimuli of the skin, joints, muscles, and inner organs) or efferent (leading away from the brain and mediating contractions of muscles or organs).

NERVOUS SYSTEM

Includes all of the neural structures in the body: The central nervous system consists of the brain, spinal cord, and optic nerves; the peripheral nervous system consists of the nerve roots and nerves throughout the body.

NEUROGENIC BLADDER

Bladder dysfunction associated with neurological malfunction in the nervous system and characterized by a failure to empty, failure to store, or a combination of the two. Symptoms that result from these three types of dysfunction include urinary urgency, frequency, hesitancy, nocturia, and incontinence.

NEUROLOGIST

Physician who specializes in the diagnosis and treatment of conditions related to the nervous system.

NEURON

The basic nerve cell of the nervous system. A neuron consists of a nucleus within a cell body and one or more processes (extensions) called dendrites and axons.

OCCUPATIONAL THERAPIST (OT)

OTs assess functioning in activities of everyday living that are essential for independent living, including dressing, bathing, grooming, meal preparation, writing, and driving. They design treatment to develop, recover, or maintain daily living or working skills.

OLIGOCLONAL BANDS

A diagnostic sign indicating abnormal levels of certain antibodies in the cerebrospinal fluid; seen in approximately 90 percent of people with MS, but not specific to MS. There are a number of procedures that can show the protein patterns in the CSF and blood and it is important to observe when the bands are seen in the CSF and are not just a reflection of the same pattern in the blood.

OLIGODENDROCYTE

A cell in the central nervous system that is responsible for making and supporting myelin.

OPTIC NEURITIS

Inflammation or demyelination of the optic (visual) nerve. It usually recovers but can leave some permanent visual change. Visual evoked potential studies can show slowed conduction in the optic nerve even when the person now feels the visual symptoms have fully recovered.

ORTHOSIS

A mechanical appliance (such as a leg brace or splint) that is specially designed to control, correct, or compensate for impaired limb function.

PARESTHESIA

A sensation of burning, prickling, or tingling on the skin that is often seen in MS.

PAROXYSMAL SYMPTOMS

Symptoms that have sudden onset, apparently in response to some kind of movement or sensory stimulation, last for a few moments, and then subside. Paroxysmal symptoms tend to occur frequently in those individuals who have them, and follow a similar pattern from one episode to the next. Examples of paroxysmal symptoms include acute episodes of trigeminal neuralgia (sharp facial pain), tonic seizures (intense spasm of limb or limbs on one side of the body), dysarthria (slurred speech often accompanied by loss of balance and coordination), and various paresthesias (sensory disturbances ranging from tingling to severe pain).

PHYSIATRIST
Physicians who specialize in the rehabilitation of physical impairments.

PHYSICAL THERAPIST, PHYSIOTHERAPIST (PT)
PTs evaluate and improve movement and function of the body, with particular attention to physical mobility, balance, posture, fatigue, and pain.

PLACEBO
An inactive compound. It is a term applied to a medicine with little or no effect but might have a positive result because of anticipation of benefit in the patient. In a clinical trial, the placebo is made to look similar to the test drug to be able to assess its benefit, safety, and limitations.

PLACEBO EFFECT
An apparently beneficial result of therapy that occurs because of the patient's expectation that the therapy will help. The placebo, which is inert, does not have the effect; it is an effect produced by the mind of the receiver.

PLAQUE
An area of inflamed or demyelinated central nervous system tissue.

POSTURAL TREMOR
Rhythmic shaking that occurs when the muscles are tensed to hold an object or stay in a given position.

PREVALENCE
The number of all new and old cases of a disease in a defined population at a particular point in time.

PRIMARY PROGRESSIVE MS

A clinical course of MS characterized from the beginning by a progressive disease.

PROGNOSIS

Prediction of the future course of the disease.

PROGRESSIVE-RELAPSING MS

A clinical course of MS that shows disease progression from the beginning, but with clear, acute relapses along the way.

PSEUDO-EXACERBATION

A temporary aggravation of disease symptoms, sometimes resulting from an elevation in body temperature or other stressor (e.g., an infection, severe fatigue, constipation), that disappears once the stressor is removed. A pseudo-exacerbation involves temporary flare-ups of prior or existing symptoms rather than new disease activity or progression.

PYRAMIDAL TRACTS

Motor nerve pathways in the brain and spinal cord that connect nerve cells in the brain to the motor cells located in the cranial, thoracic, and lumbar parts of the spinal cord. Damage to these tracts causes spastic paralysis or weakness.

REFLEX

An involuntary response of the nervous system to a stimulus, such as the stretch reflex, which is elicited by tapping a tendon with a reflex hammer, resulting in a contraction. Increased, diminished, or absent reflexes can be indicative of neurological damage, including MS, and are therefore tested as part of the standard neurological exam.

RELAPSE

Also known as an attack, flare-up, or exacerbation. The appearance of new symptoms or the aggravation of old ones, lasting at least 24 hours; usually associated with inflammation and demyelination in the brain or spinal cord.

RELAPSING-REMITTING MS

A clinical course of MS that is characterized by clearly defined, acute attacks (relapses) with full or partial recovery and no disease progression between attacks.

REMISSION

A lessening in the severity of symptoms or their temporary disappearance during the course of the illness.

REMYELINATION

The repair of damaged myelin. Myelin repair occurs spontaneously in MS but the new myelin is thinner and conducts a little more slowly.

SCLEROSIS

Hardening or scarring of tissue. In MS, sclerosis is the replacement of lost myelin around central nervous system nerve cells with scar tissue.

SECONDARY PROGRESSIVE MS

A clinical course of MS that initially is relapsing-remitting and then becomes progressive at a variable rate, with or without occasional relapses along the way. The disease-modifying medications are thought to provide benefit for those who continue to have relapses.

SENSORY

Related to bodily sensations such as pain, smell, taste, temperature, vision, hearing, and position in space.

SIGN

An objective physical problem or abnormality identified by the physician during the neurological examination, including altered eye movements and other changes in the appearance or function of the visual system; altered reflexes; weakness; spasticity; and sensory changes.

SPASTICITY

Abnormal increase in muscle tone, manifested as a springlike resistance of an extremity to moving or being moved.

SPHINCTER

A circular band of muscle fibers that tightens or closes a natural opening of the body, such as the external anal sphincter, which closes the anus, and the internal and external urinary sphincters, which close the urinary canal.

SPINAL TAP

See Lumbar puncture

STEROIDS

See Glucocorticoid hormones.

SYMPTOM

A subjectively perceived problem or complaint reported by the patient. In MS, common symptoms include visual problems, fatigue, sensory changes, weakness or paralysis of the limbs, tremor, lack of coordination, poor balance, bladder or bowel changes, and psychological changes. *See* Sign.

TONIC SEIZURE

An intense spasm that lasts for a few minutes and affects one or both limbs on one side of the body. Like other types of paroxysmal symptoms in MS, these spasms occur abruptly and fairly frequently in those individuals who have them, and are similar from one brief episode to the next. The attacks may be triggered by movement or occur spontaneously. *See* Paroxysmal symptom.

TRIGEMINAL NEURALGIA

Lightning-like, stabbing acute pain in the face caused by demyelination of nerve fibers at the site where the sensory (trigeminal) nerve root for that part of the face enters the brainstem.

URINARY FREQUENCY

Need or urge to urinate more frequently than normal due to small hyperactive bladder.

URINARY HESITANCY

The inability to void urine spontaneously even though the urge to do so is present.

URINARY URGENCY

The inability to postpone urination once the need to void has been felt.

VERTIGO

A dizzying sensation of the environment spinning, often accompanied by nausea and vomiting.

Additional Readings

There are many books with information about MS. Some are scientific, some educational, some give advice about management of various symptoms and some of therapies people are putting forward, and others are personal experiences of people with MS. It can be bewildering—Amazon has over 75 books on MS currently for sale. This is a brief list of helpful books:

Books from Demos Medical Publishing on MS

Rae-Grant A. et al. 2013. *Multiple Sclerosis and Related Disorders (Second Edition forthcoming in 2018).*

Bowling, A. 2014. *Optimal Health with Multiple Sclerosis: A Guide to Integrating Lifestyle, Alternative, and Conventional Medicine*

Bowling, A. 2007. *Complementary and Alternative Medicine and Multiple Sclerosis.*

Kalb, R. 2012. *Multiple Sclerosis: The Questions You Have, the Answers You Need, Fifth Edition.*

Murray, T. J. 2005. *Multiple Sclerosis: The History of a Disease.*

Saunders, C. 2011. *What Nurses Know … Multiple Sclerosis.*

Schwartz, S. 2017. *Multiple Sclerosis: Tips and Strategies for Making Life Easier, Third Edition.*

Shenkman, M. 2009. *Estate Planning for People With Chronic Disease.*

Other References

Marcia Finlayson. 2012. *Multiple Sclerosis Rehabilitation: From Impairment to Participation.* CRC Press.

Barbara Giesser. 2016. *Primer on Multiple Sclerosis, Second Edition.* Oxford University Press.

Dennis Greenberger and Christine Padesky. Mind over mood. 2015. *Change How You Feel by Changing the Way You Think, Second Edition.* Guilford Press.

Alirenza Minagar. 2015. *Multiple Sclerosis: A Mechanistic View,* Academic Press.

Catherine Edward. 2008. *The Brow of Dawn: One Woman's Journey With MS.* Bunim and Berigan.

Resources

There are many resources available to help you meet the challenges of multiple sclerosis. This list is by no means complete; it is designed as a starting point in your efforts to identify the resources you need. Each resource will lead to others.

Information Sources

National Health Information Center (P.O. Box 1133, Washington, DC 20013; Tel: 800-336-4797; Internet: www.health.gov/nhic). The Center maintains a library and a database of health-related organizations. It also provides referrals related to health issues for consumers and professionals.

Agencies and Organizations

National Multiple Sclerosis Society (NMSS) (733 Third Avenue, New York, NY 10017; Tel: 800-FIGHT-MS; Internet: www .nationalmsssociety.org). The NMSS is a nonprofit organization that supports national and international research into the prevention, cure, and treatment of MS. The Society's goals include provision of nationwide services to assist people with MS and their families, and provision of information to those with MS, their families, professionals, and the public. The programs and services of the Society promote knowledge, health, and independence while providing education and emotional support:

- Toll-free access by calling 800-FIGHT-MS (800-344-4867).

- Website with updated information about treatments, current research, and programs (http://www.-nationalmssociety.org); local home page in many areas.

- Knowledge Is Power—an eight-segment, learn-at-home program (serial mailings) for people newly diagnosed with MS and their families.

- MS Learn Online—online, interactive web casts on a wide variety of topics.

- Printed materials on a variety of topics available by calling 800-FIGHT-MS (800-344-4867) or in the Library section of the National Multiple Sclerosis Society website at http://www.-nationalmssociety.org/library.asp.

- Educational programs on various topics throughout the year, provided through individual chapters.

- Annual national education conference, provided through individual chapters.

- Swimming and other exercise programs sponsored or cosponsored by some chapters, or referral to existing programs in the community.

- Wellness programs in some chapters.

Multiple Sclerosis Society of Canada (250 Bloor Street East, Suite 100, Toronto, ON, M4W 3P9 Canada; Tel 416-922-6065; in

Canada: 800-268-7582; Internet: www.mssociety.ca). A national organization that funds research, promotes public education, and produces publications in both English and French. They provide an "ASK MS Information System" database of articles on a wide variety of topics including treatment, research, and social services. Regional divisions and chapters are located throughout Canada.

Consortium of Multiple Sclerosis Centers (CMSC) (c/o 59 Main Street, Suite A, Hackensack, NJ 07601; Tel: 201-487-1050, Internet: www.mscare.org). The CMSC is made up of numerous MS centers throughout the United States and Canada. The Consortium's mission is to disseminate information to clinicians, increase resources and opportunities for research, and advance the standard of care for MS. The CMSC is a multidisciplinary organization, bringing together health care professionals from many fields involved in MS patient care.

Department of Veterans Affairs (VA) (810 Vermont Avenue, N.W., Washington, DC 20420; Tel: 202-273-5400; Internet: www. va.gov). The VA provides a wide range of benefits and services to those who have served in the armed forces, their dependents, beneficiaries of deceased veterans, and dependent children of veterans with severe disabilities.

Equal Employment Opportunity Commission (EEOC) (Office of Communication and Legislative Affairs, 1801 L Street, N.W., 10th Floor, Washington, DC 20507; Tel: 800-669-3362 (to order publications); 800-669-4000 (to speak to an investigator); 202-663-4900; Internet: www.eeoc.gov). The EEOC is responsible for monitoring the section of the Americans with Disabilities Act (ADA) on employment regulations. Copies of the regulations are available.

Can Do MS (27 Main St., Suite 303, Edwards, CO 81632; Tel; 1-800-367-3101; Internet: http://www.mscando.org). Can Do MS is a non-profit organization dedicated to improving the lives of people and families living with MS through interactive, educational programs unique to any in the world. With an interdisciplinary team of MS experts in fields such as neurology; psychology; occupational, physical, and speech therapy; and nutrition, the CAN DO,

JUMPSTART, and other Can Do MS programs offer a supportive, nurturing environment in which participants learn to take control of their lives and their health by focusing on what they "can do" instead of what they cannot. The Center's programs, offered throughout North America, help participants set realistic personal goals, construct an individualized lifestyle plan, and gain the strategies and skills necessary to be successful in improving their lives. Can Do MS programs also address the needs and education of support partners and family members.

United Spinal Association (USA) (75-20 Astoria Boulevard, Jackson Heights, NY 11370; Tel: 718-803-3782; Internet: www .unitedspinal.org). USA is a private, nonprofit organization dedicated to serving the needs of its members as well as other people with spinal cord injury or disorder. While offering a wide range of benefits to members with spinal cord dysfunction (including hospital liaison, sports and recreation, wheelchair repair, adaptive architectural consultations, research and educational services, communications, and information services), they will also provide brochures and information on a variety of subjects, free of charge to the general public.

Well Spouse Foundation (610 Lexington Avenue, New York, NY 10022-6005; Tel: 212-644-1241; 800-838-0879; Internet: www. wellspouse.org). An emotional support network for people married to or living with a chronically ill partner. Advocacy for home health and long-term care and a newsletter are among the services offered.

Electronic Information Sources

There are many sources of information available free through the Internet on the world wide web. If you are an experienced "net surfer," switch to your favorite search facility and enter the keywords "MS" or "multiple sclerosis." This will generally give you a listing of dozens of websites that pertain to MS. Keep in mind, however, that the world wide web is a free and open medium; while many of the websites have excellent and useful information, others may contain highly unusual and inaccurate information. A good place to start ...

Complete Drug Reference (Compiled by United States Pharmacopoeia, published by Consumer Report Books, A division of Consumers Union, Yonkers, NY.) This comprehensive, readable, and easy-to-use drug reference includes almost every prescription and non-prescription medication available in the United States and Canada. A new edition is published yearly.

Index

About the Author

T. Jock Murray, OC, ONS, MD, FRCPC, MACP, FAAN, FRCP, MCFP, FCAHS (Honorary LLD, DSc, DFA, D.Litt, LLD)

Dr. T. Jock Murray is professor emeritus of Medicine and Neurology and former Dean of Medicine at Dalhousie University in Halifax, Nova Scotia, Canada. He served as president of the Canadian Neurological Society, vice president of the American Academy of Neurology and two terms as chairman of the American College of Physicians. Although he has international awards for his contributions to medical education, medical history, and medical administration, his clinical and research devotion was always to patients with multiple sclerosis. He has published over three hundred medical papers, held ninety-one funded research grants and authored eight books and forty-eight book chapters. He was a founder of the Consortium of MS Centers and the Canadian Network of MS Centers, and was awarded the Dr. Labe Scheinberg Award for contributions to MS research. His publication of *Multiple Sclerosis: The History of a Disease*, was awarded the ForeWord Silver Medal as the best book on history in 2005. He has been awarded five honorary degrees, the Order of Nova Scotia and is an Officer of the Order of Canada. In 2014 he was elected to the Canadian Medical Hall of Fame. He is proudest of his wife, Janet, who contributed in a huge way to all of the above, and his four children and seven grandchildren.